Dr. med. Hans-Peter Greb

The true Walk

From heeling to healing

The dynamic Yoga GODO

Prevent Backaches and Postural Defects &
Things to know about Natural Walking

Translated from German
by Ruth Bleakley-Thiessen

Illustrations by Lucie Deinzer

The original first edition was published in Germany under the title "GODO – Mit dem Herzen gehen. Der Gang des neuen Menschen" in KOHA Verlag in 2000.

The fifth edition was published under the title "Ballengang: Rückenschmerzen und Haltungsschäden vorbeugen – Wissenswertes über das natürliche Gehen".

Copyright: © 2018 Hans-Peter Greb
From German into English: Ruth Bleakley-Thiessen

Publisher:
Verlag und Druck:
tredition GmbH
Halenreie 40-44
22359 Hamburg

All rights reserved. No part of this publication may be reproduced, translated, distributed, or transmitted in any form or by any means, including photocopying, recording, or other electronic or mechanical methods, without the prior written permission of the publisher and author.

The disclosed recommendations in this book have been carefully processed and verified by the author.
A gaurantee can nevertheless not be issued. Similarly the author is excluded from any liability for personal, material and financial damage.

I dedicate this book to

Mic Dodge
THE BAREFOOT SENSEI
my brother in the wilderhood

Content

Introduction 7
My Journey with GODO 13
First Scientific Proof 18
The Human is a Ball-Gaiter 25
   Experience as a Doctor 25
Second Scientific Proof: 27
   The Stepping Reflex 28
   The First Steps 29
   The Behaviour of Imitation 30
The Walking Performance of the Human 33
   The Platonic Soul Skills and GODO 33
   Resting 34
   Wanting 35
   Thinking 35
   Gait Analysis 37
   The Gestures of the Heel-walk 38
   So-called Marching on the Spot and Military Marching 41
The Gestures of the Ball-gait 44
   Feeling 44
   Coming to Rest 45
   Me-Strength 46
   From Thinking to Thanking 47
   Gait and ME-development 49
   Fear of Falling, Ego and Superego 55
   The SELF 58
   Circulation, Emotional Body and Gender Emancipation 59
   Research and Insights through Observation 65
Third Scientific Proof: 68
Fourth Scientific Proof: 71
   What about Indigenous People? 73

Evolution **76**
   Reptilian Brain and the Heel Bone 76
   Gait and Language 79

Pregnancy, Birth and the "Sensitive Phase" **83**
   Regular Birth, Power – Powerlessness, Defiant Behaviour, Sexist
   Socialisation 87
   Water Birth 92
   The Aquatic Ape 99

Feet, Fashion and GODO **103**
   Lotus Feet 103
   The History of Heel Fashion 105

How do I learn GODO quickest? **108**
   As a Ball-Gaiter you will become the Person you are 108
   The New Footwear... 110
   Now to the Practice ….. 111

The Practical Success of GODO **117**
   GODO Fitness 120

A Report based on Experience out of my Practice **122**
   The Miraculous Healing of an Eight-year-old Boy 122

Experiences with GODO **128**
   Out of my GODO Diary.. 128
   The Experience of Oneness in Walking 130
   Readers' Letters 131

On Walking **149**

Closing Words **156**

The Training Course to become a GODOLOGIST **158**

Acknowledgements **161**

Bibliography **162**

Introduction

Your first steps ... do you still remember them?
Or ... do you feel them within you?
Think about it!
It was the unique getting up and going out into the world ...
out ... up and run.
A ME opening itself to the world,
just rapturously traipsing out of yourself ...
weightless, completely indulged, saying, "Yees, yeess!" –
and then the first flops onto the floor, letting yourself be drawn up again,
having become centred, out of and into everything that comes ...
stays ... is,
and having vibrant willingness
for ever new ecstasies.

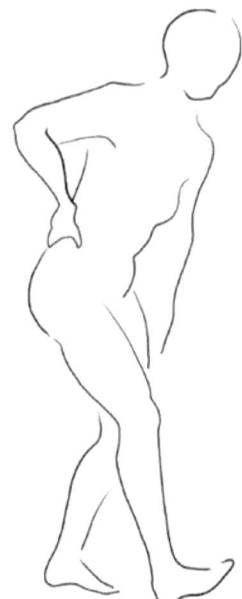

From heeling …

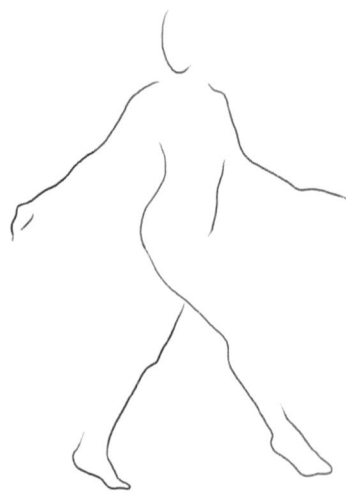

… to healing.

Having founded the "Institute for applied Humane Morphology" in 1979 and the "GODO Walking School", which is connected to it, I held countless workshops and lectures and trained seventy GODOLOGISTs, who are authorised to spread the message about GODO in Germany, Austria, Switzerland, Luxembourg and Italy, in the USA and most recently in Venezuela and Paraguay as well. My television appearance in 2001 in Germany with Alfred Biolek certainly whet the appetite of several million people within a short time for a new feeling of life.

Now this book has been published in the fifth edition in Germany. In 1974 I discovered that the human being is genetically a forefoot-walker: therefore, walking on the forefoot, the ball-gait, is our natural way of walking and not the commonly practised treading on the heel, which is held for normal.

From the medical side there has been no such awareness of this fact before, not to mention a name for it. The international medical field only knows the descriptions and terms of walking disorders. Therefore I had to give my discovery of the natural forefoot-gait an internationally valid name: GODO.

GODO has meanwhile become the topic of many holistic-thinking doctors and physiotherapists – and is even recognised as further education for medical doctors.

The source of GODO is neatly quoted in the physio-therapeutic dissertation of Mathias Hofbauer and in the GODO Training Manual from Dirk Beckmann as "simple ball-gait – natural gait". As a fascia therapist, the latter applies the ball-gait to help people in pain to a better, more erect body structure. As he says, it is "the more intelligent of these contemporaries". Free-runners, retro-runners and barefoot-walkers also discovered the ball-gait with GODO and joyfully describe their reanimated body intelligence and agility.

In contrast, you can find clips about forefoot-runners, such as Professor Daniel E. Lieberman, practising barefoot-jogging through New York. He explains the gentle, physiologically efficient, softly cushioned step used exclusively for running/jogging. Doctrinally committed medical professionals like him weren't able to comprehend the logical conclusion up until now, that the ball-gait is our natural, inherent bipedal program for movement. This explains many injuries runners always get when they change over to forefoot running, being poorly trained without walking/striding on the forefoot.

By the way, in the German language, the meaning of "walking" (as in *gehen*) and "walking" (as in *laufen*) is continuously mixed-up in different areas. This book should finally clear the problem about the meaning of the term, and will take the proverbial "bandages off the eyes" of the dogmatically biased orthodox medical practitioners on the issue of the heel-walk. The program heel-walk, which we unfortunately seem to have installed into our heads, shoots consistent interfering patterns into our extra-pyramidal, genetically designed, natural motional patterns in walking or running. Perhaps even reflexively into our thoughts and the verbal expression thereof, which manifest as an imbalance of context. That could be the deeper reason that forefoot-runners, such as Dr Ulrich Strunz, Dr Matthias Marquardt, Dr Thomas Wessinghage or Professor Daniel Lieberman, still always mistreat themselves with the heel-walk.

My unreserved recognition is found only in whoever entirely stands his claim to GODO, for GODO isn't just a ball-gait. Whoever talks or writes about the ball-gait without mentioning the term GODO, or when a person doesn't quote my name together with GODO, withholds large parts of the scientific meaning of GODO and makes an unauthorised simplification of it, as well as being guilty of plagiarism in an exemption of the meaning of it. You find a lot of such imitators on the internet, who advertise themselves as therapists and amongst other things, selling shoes, and can be found under searchwords like "forefoot-walking", "natural gait", "ball-walk" or "barefoot-walk".

Thankfully, a lot has changed since I first outed myself in public as the first discoverer of the scientifically proven fact that human beings are genetically inherent ball-gaiters. In the meantime I am pleased about the approval the ball-gait now experiences. Today reports of progress come in daily from forefoot-gaiters, who have encountered my message. They are happy about the disappearance of varicose veins; they report that they have never twisted their ankle again; after they discovered GODO, they suffered less from slipped discs and a lot of pain in the knee, hip and feet disappeared. All of them feel enriched and share their good experiences with others.

This book is the result of a consequent, interdisciplinary research, in which I followed my longing for an absolute body consciousness and the wish to understand my feet. At first I thought I had to use a lot of persuasion and sneer at the heel-walkers in order to startle them so that they would understand me. Now I know that we only need a small impulse to remember that we are ball-gaiters from the time of birth. So I have "polished" my book and expanded it with various testimonies.

If you like, I'll take you on a journey with me, on which you can get to know your natural way of walking. You will remember your wholeness by striding naturally over the balls of the feet, which is common to all human beings. Perhaps you will get a new feeling for yourself, as so many GODO supporters have done. It is an exciting experience, an exciting journey – also to yourself. I cordially invite you to go on this journey. I wish you lots of joy and insights in reading this book, and naturally with GODO!

My Journey with GODO

*"Anybody who walks consciously and alertly,
not only discovers an exterior world,
but himself at the same time."*

Markus Dederich:
In the order of the Body (In den Ordnungen des Leibes)

Let me take you on a journey of letting go an unnecessary, absurd practice of walking. Ever since we learnt to walk by imitation, we have wearily been practising it all over the whole world. It's about a silent revolt, overcoming a way of walking we have become accustomed to everywhere, it's about letting go in the ankle joint, which in German is called the *"Fessel"*, and can be translated as the "chain". So it's all about breaking free from your chains, and liberating yourself.

By way of introduction here's a story I have for you:
I recently walked through a park and overtook, despite my unhurried pace, an approximately seventy-year-old woman who was walking arduously. She looked around several times, so that our eyes met dead on as I was level with her. I sensed that she wanted to smile back at me, but pain held her features captive, and in the same moment she was on the verge of falling over a small stone. Reflexively, I caught her upper arm, and both of us came to a halt. It sputtered out of her: "Thanks!" Her face relaxed. "Yes, I can still stand without pain, but you know, I have a heel spur and since getting the new hip I have the old sciatic pain now and again that everything started with. I've just come from physiotherapy and have to learn to

properly roll off from the heel of my foot, and it's exactly that which is extremely painful."

I asked her if she walked at home without shoes.

"Yes, it's all different there! I take tiny little steps, and then it's okay. But I can't walk about like that. What would it look like?!"

Now I had my cue. She already knew the solution! I didn't need to recommend a new way of walking to her, instead I asked her just to walk as she did at home.

She looked around to see that no one was watching. We were alone – she scuttled on. I was hardly able to keep up with her, her movement was so in flow, and she began to giggle. "You see, but what does it look like?!" She had stopped herself already, and her features once again fell into pain.

"Become like a small child!" I heard a voice inside of me. And I began to tell her about GODO, the healthy gait of human beings.

Meanwhile we had reached the lawn beside the path. We had taken off our shoes and enjoyed the cool grass. We rolled off from the top of the foot (toes and ball) onto the heel – she had no pain any more. Her walk was like that of a queen again, and if you believe it or not: she looked twenty years younger!

If you also long for such a wonderful experience, then read on. I'm taking you on a journey to the source of your natural health and vitality.

Do you remember the first scuttling steps of your child? It ran quite easily over the balls of its feet to you. With its little arms upraised, it seemed to want to take off like an airplane. And do you also remember your fear watching your child losing balance and falling? You ran towards it or after it, quickly took it into your arms, and in doing so – unknowing of course and acting for its own best – unsettled it in its spontaneous, inbred, healthy, natural walk over the balls of its feet, for small children live in the emotional protective shield of the mother and feel her uncertainty.

Seemingly effortlessly the little ones balance their large head on a stretched spine. We were born with a stretched spine. Up until the first steps walking on the heels it is bolt upright and for this reason maximally flexible in all of its joints. The small body achieved all movements skilfully and without effort. This is only possible because of an efficient genetic program of movement. It is born as a ball-gaiter. But from the first year of life, together with the acquisition of speech, it mutates by imitation to a heel-walker!

In fact we are all ball-gaiters. What we were never really conscious of, will be made conscious to us for the first time here in this book. It is the memory of an ancient right of birth, that has been forgotten for the last five million years.

The practical success of GODO lies in comprehensive rehabilitation and health care. In the process, GODO not only leads to superficial wellness and fitness, rather it goes as far as the depths of inner and outer ecology. GODO could enable us to let the world become a paradise again, simply by admitting to ourselves what we actually are, namely ball-gaiters.

Today ninety-nine per cent of all people walk through life on their heels. We have become accustomed to imitating walking the wrong way. We march with a thrust of the heel onto the earth. We abuse our feet and all of our joints with an inefficient landing on the heel, and suffer the consequences of this self-abuse with bad posture and pain.

What we do to ourselves with every step on the heel not only has an impact on the body, mind and soul, but also on our social reality. Love your neighbour as you love yourself. The quality of the love you have for yourself is the level on which you are able to love others. The heel-walk is a lie of movement, the effects of which are more alarming and worldwide important than we can sense. Kicking our ass in every step is desensitising ourselves to a degree we had better become conscious of, before we can begin to realise the effects of it. Currently we are confronted with xenophobia (racism and hatred of foreigners), which could also be generalised as the fascism in each of us. Who's kicking me in the behind? In French it's called: I'm madly annoyed = *je suis faché*. In German it can be translated as: I am sour. Are not all heel-walkers necessarily tending to be *faché* in the depth of their unconsciousness?

For me, this book is about more than just criticism on the shoe industry, which wants to sell us wellness-barefoot-walking with capping (cages in front of the feet), heels (shots), pads and cushions for the heels, arch supports, and since 1996, rolling, round shoes. In reality we are buying "artificial limbs" for ourselves and then we ask ourselves why we get postural deformities, back pain, circulation problems, vein complaints and the foot complaints already mentioned. All that is being *faché,* is like feeling sick. But as every one of us is harming himself the same way with the heel-walk, we are all living in a mad house, where the doctor has lost the key.

Prostheses are only needed when we have to restore a lost function. Every application of prostheses on a healthy body leads to the suppression and the loss of functions. So, what are we doing to ourselves here?!

As a doctor and a humane morphologist (human gestalt investigator), during many years of experience in my practice, I watched and researched the walking performance of my patients. The practice of walking on the heel creates jolting which reaches up into the skull.

First Scientific Proof:

An impressive phrasing of that which we require as scientific proof is provided by Jutta Voss in her book *"Das Schwarzmond-Tabu"* (The Black Moon Taboo):

"I owe everything to "looking", which in Buddhism is an essential exercise of meditation, that also includes the empirical aspect of the repeatable. [...] Looking is the foundation of knowledge. The knowledge of wisdom is impossible without looking at inquiry. All knowledge has its origin in looking at reality, how it is and how it essentially is."

With a practical exercise, you can easily become aware of what the heel-walk does to you: put your fingers into your ears and walk ten to twenty steps quickly in your normal manner. In doing so, listen inside yourself! Did you hear it, this tock-tock-tock? You have herewith given yourself scientific proof, repeatable at any time (see the chapter on "The Gestures of the Heel-walk").

I came to the conclusion that in the way people walk – that is to say: upright–walking, we should first of all bring the forefoot to the ground with each step, in order to then sink the heel down. In this way we touch the earth feather-light and save ourselves from the shock in our spine up into our head. So it's exactly the opposite of all the orthopaedic recommendations!

Eighty-five per cent of our fellow citizens suffer from complaints of poor posture. That's no wonder, because already eighty-five per cent of preschool children (!) show severe postural deformities.

Frequent illnesses resulting from these postural deformities are common to a large extent, with pain in the bones, joints and muscles. How many of us haven't at some time already had hollow feet, splayfeet, flatfeet or abducted feet pointed out by a doctor, if we complained about some pain in the feet, knees, hips or back? Many were prescribed insoles or were at least recommended them. How often were they of no help, or provided only temporary relief? Usually you were simply encouraged to believe that you brought an inherited disposition with you when you came into the world, which could get worse over the years.

Due to foot-beds and insoles, that the shoe industry promotes as "supporting, carrying, or holding" the foot, we are spoon-fed out of our shoes and on top of it debilitated with shoes which are too narrow and too firm. On the other hand, as the saying goes: bullied around. In comparison to this GODO, or the art of the ball-gait, treading, is the ideal way to get strong, "awakened" feet. This has been demonstrated to us up until now by many people practising GODO.

The muscles in our forefoot send signals to the brain and after that on to the whole body, about how it can straighten up in perfect, self-regulating balance. All of our intrinsic muscles, which lie close around the spine, cater for an elastic straightening and a self-confident, self-assured stance. The muscles in our forefoot signal the state of the ground to us when stepping sensitively. The "awakened" feet make us attentive to ourselves, so that we can avoid and counterbalance possible poor postures as early as the origin of the root cause.

When we humans are happy, when we express pleasure, don't we lift ourselves all on our own up onto the forefoot – or as we call it:

the balls of the feet? As in dancing, we feel light, and a feeling of well-being flows through us. With the ball-gait, the whole body stretches itself. We breathe more freely; we have the feeling of breathing with the whole body, and our feeling of healthy self-worth becomes considerably stronger.

We all suspect that there is something going "wrong" with us, and everyone asks: "How's it going?" To make matters worse, the doctors recommend the so-called "proper rolling off" to us. This rolling off is probably the most dangerous medical dogma. It commits us all to heel-walking. (A dogma is an unproven accepted claim, a belief with the demand of implicit importance. With Jutta Voss it sounds like this: "[…] unquestionable and specified as the only valid truth since the beginning of the world […]. It is imperative to believe in it, no matter if experience and knowledge show the opposite.")

Having found a name that can be understood globally for the retrieved fact that we are genetically set up as ball-gaiters, I came upon the pun GODO. It consists of the syllables GO and DO. GO is the name of the oldest game in the world; it comes from Japan and means "**through playing to awareness**". DO as in "Aikido" or "Judo" means "the road". In English "go, do" is the request: "Go and do! Move and act!"

With that we mean: "**Walk the road consciously!**"

In Italian "godo" means: "I enjoy". As in "*mi godo la vita*" – "I enjoy life".

And since Samuel Beckett's play *Waiting for Godo(t)* are we not all waiting? There, in similar form, it's repeatedly called:

Estragon: *Allons-nous-en. Come, we're going.*
Vladimir: *On ne peut pas. We can't.*
Estragon: *Pourquoi? Why?*
Vladimir: *On attend Godot. We're waiting on Godot.*
Or somewhat further into the play:
Estragon: *Et s'il vient? And if he comes?*
Vladimir: *Nous serons sauvés. Then we are saved.*

It's an interesting visionary statement which Beckett made there in the second half of the year 1945, when he wrote that piece.

GODO teaches us how we can properly walk upright over the balls of the feet. In doing so, a harmonic sequence of motion is developed, which produces these following gestures:

resting
wanting
thanking/thinking
feeling
coming to rest
resting

The heel-walk, on the other hand, has an impaired motional procedure with the consequence of the following gestures (see the chapter "The Walking Performance of the Human"):

wanting
thinking instead of thanking
not wanting to feel and not wanting to want

The contradictory motor driven control of the feet in the heel-walk (wanting – not wanting) influences the carriage of the spine, the breath, and the circulation, and it causes severe mis-connections in the brain, which are to be taken seriously.

The fact that the development of walking and talking not only takes place parallel to each other in the first three years of our life, but they also use the same nerve cords, can cause a failure of expression and meaning (see the chapter on "Gait and Language").

The human being is press-ganged from being a ball-gaiter into a heel-walker by the early process of adjustment, the so-called learning of walking, and due to this, was brought out of harmony not only physically, but also mentally. We are therefore, impaired, so to speak! (Note from translator: in German: the author wrote "*gehstört*", which literally translated means impaired in walking.) We have been trained into a distorted disguise of movement by the imitation of a false example, the heel-walk. We have learnt marching instead of gaiting.

Many poor postures, which haven't been caused by an accident, an injury, or through genetic defects, I ascribe to the heel-walk more than anything else. Furthermore, in the course of this book, it will be made clear how much inhumane regular birth has confused our mobility right from the start. In addition, the benefits of the water birth in unfolding our natural movement will be presented in detail.

GODO is also more than a forefoot gait. GODO informs about possibilities to sensitively connect with the earth, to see a living being in her and lovingly experience yourself, step by step, in straightening to an upright body posture. By walking more consciously, we also live more consciously. In dynamic straightening doing striding, ball-emphasised forward movement, we unfold our purest Me, because:

The ME is the upright body posture!

Only a ball-emphasised use of the feet can lead to a perfect straightening up (see the chapter "Gait and ME-development")!

The basic principles of what has been described here have been known in detail for a long time. To retrieve them and to put the pieces back together serves the awakening and the confirmation of common memory.

Feel for yourself how the new, or rather, the rediscovered way of walking creates a soothing strength in the whole organism when you reawaken to it by striding normally on the balls of the feet. You will be amazed.

The neurologist Prof. Gerald Huether from Goettingen calls the delight *"doping for mind and brain"*. And further:
"Unfortunately grown-ups can only occasionally remember their first childhood experiences. Remember this feeling of happiness, with which you set out as a small child to explore the world. You can hardly remember this unbelievable openness, this desire to create and the joy of discovery. You only have a clouded notion of this enthusiasm for yourself and for everything there was to discover and to make flowing through the whole body. If these memories were more present, many worries, problems and hardships of adulthood wouldn't exist."

The summary of positive effects on your health can be found in the chapter on "The Practical Success of GODO". Seemingly negative effects – I call that healing pains - are of a temporary nature and apart from that, are seldom. Only in the first days of transition to the ball-gait you will have some sore muscles, mostly in the calves. That's very instructive for the beginner, because he notices where he was insufficiently challenged up until now.

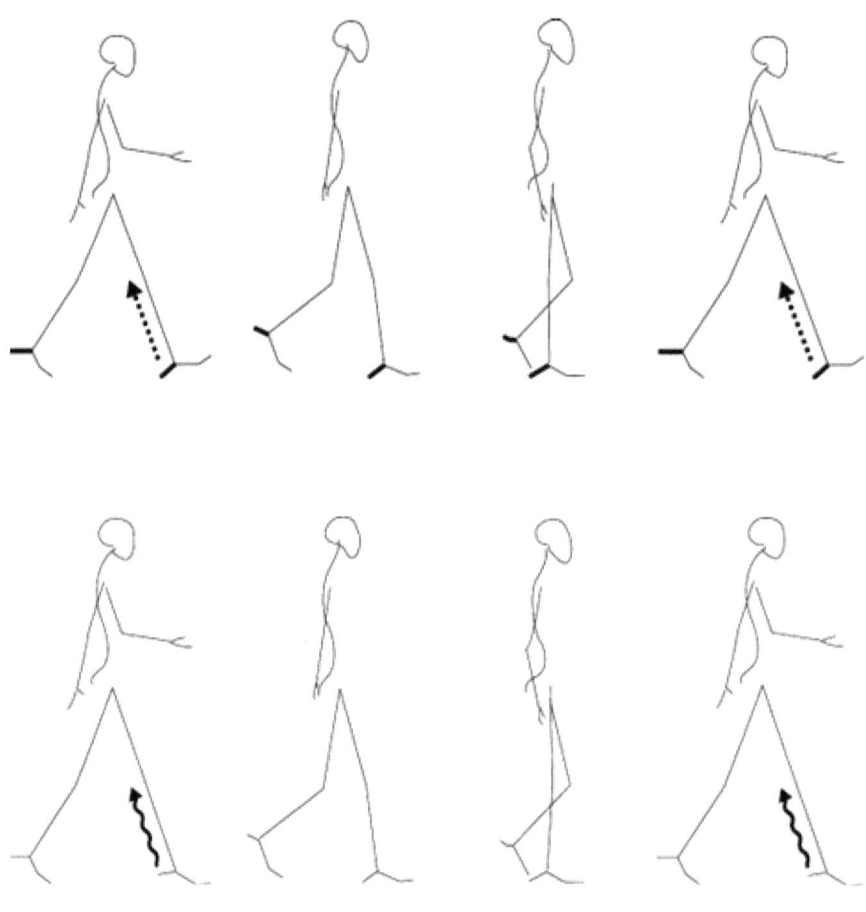

The Human is a Ball-Gaiter

Experience as a Doctor

In my work on the symptoms of pain in the muscular and the skeletal system, it struck me at the start of my medical work (in the beginning of the Seventies), that humans probably unnecessarily afflict themselves with their walking pattern.

The discovery that the human being is actually a ball-gaiter began with an accidental observation, which caused me to assume that the medicine I learned, was literally on the wrong track. I was seized by great doubt, and only in-depth research and stubborn clinging to my discovery has made this book possible. Last but not least, my now around forty-five-year-long self-experiment of going through life in the ball-gait has given me the courage to recommend you to do the same.

How did I come across these insights in the first place? In my first consulting room there was a huge baroque mirror that was built into the wall of the sixty square metre large consulting room. In front of it was the treatment table. After I wrote down the medical history, I accompanied my patient straight across the room to the mirror. In order to estimate the structural symptoms of my patient better, I observed the symmetry of their sequence of movement. In doing so, my hand glided over their back to discover eventual tenseness, which shows up in a difference in temperature.

In order to improve my sensibility, I took off my shoes. In doing so, I was able to move so quietly, that I could perceive the finest vibrations and the compensatory muscular contractions of my patients.

As different as the signs were which pointed out to the individual suffering, so clearly was the strong "tock-tock" felt with all of them, to a lesser or greater extent. This "tock" came from the impact of the heel, with which we, as heel-walkers, all tread on the earth. It could be felt especially well in laying a hand on the sacral bone of the person being examined, whilst he walked quite normally. Try this some time with a fellow human being. This rates as …

Second Scientific Proof:

In order to be able to walk quietly and observantly beside them, I unconsciously began to walk over the forefoot myself. After some months, on the way home in the evening, I heard my own heel-walking steps, the "tock-tock-tock" ringing out on the walls of the houses as an echo. I was horrified. Awakened by the shock, I began to assume that the ball-gait is the gait which corresponds to our true nature.

After I had consciously observed the mindfulness and the lightness of the ball-gait, the heel-walk seemed to me to be a very rough method of movement. I began to realise that the heel-walk could be the cause of most bad postures and the resulting pain in the muscular and skeletal system.

I asked myself why we don't move with more feeling in our daily life, hence with the emphasis on the balls of the feet. Our aesthetic ideals even invite it! Just think of high-heels, dance, ballet, walking training for models, the position of the feet on dummies in shop windows and "stepping the royal gait". Even the common use of language shows us a feeling that boundaries can be CROSSED (in German it is *Überschreiten* = stride over), but should never be IGNORED.

Furthermore, we jump on bouncy feet when we are happy, whilst we express anger by stamping on the ground with the heel of the foot. And whoever doesn't use the spring-force of the feet in sport, isn't able to perform well and looks inelegant, even clumsy.

On top of that it struck me that people who moved a lot, e.g. danced freely in the club, seldom came to my practice. On the other hand, I often had to treat professional dancers with their typical wear and tear and sport injuries. In the course of time it became clear to me, that these were mostly only the consequences of artificially trained and exaggerated poor posture, caused by the impact of the strike of the heels.

So I asked myself:

Why are we WALKING on our heels?
Why are we not STRIDING over the balls of our feet?

The Stepping Reflex

For this reason I began to interest myself for the development of the human pattern of movement in a new way, and I turned to the origin of the development of our walking. Right from the beginning I observed children from the moment of their birth. In doing so, the first thing I noticed was the medically so-called stepping reflex of newborns. I want to call it "gait reflex" and not "stepping reflex", because it has to do with an explicit movement, with the emphasis on the balls of the feet. This reflex can normally only be observed within a limited period of time in all babies, namely from the time of birth up until the age of four to six weeks. By the way, this reflex is maintained by those born under water up until they learn to walk very early in the sixth month (more about that in the chapter on "Pregnancy, Birth and the "Sensitive Phase"").

Everyone who has held a child under a year old in his arms whilst sitting down, notices that the child presses with the tips of its feet into your stomach. It is quite natural that it does this with the sensitive forefoot and not with the heel. Furthermore, I noticed how small the heel of a newborn is.

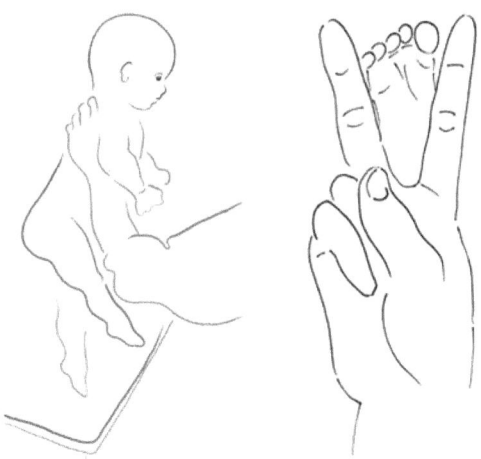

See for yourself how unsuitable the heel is for the heel walk

The First Steps

Next I noticed that all children taking their first steps are obviously still distinct ball-gaiters. Every father and mother will confirm that. It can only escape our attention if we dress the child right from the start in shoes with stiff soles, and don't allow it to walk barefoot often enough.

I observed that children under three years old became ball-gaiters again if they moved to-

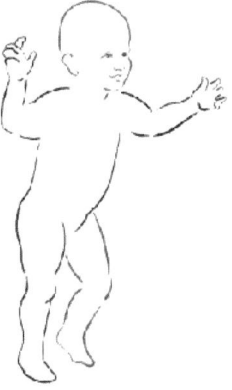

wards something very interesting. In such moments they feel themselves unobserved. However, as long as they feel themselves being observed, they try as well as possible to imitate the heel-walk. I thus asked myself the question: do children become heel-walkers because they want to walk exactly like their parents?

The Behaviour of Imitation

Psychology teaches about the imitating behaviour of children, that they almost exclusively learn by imitation in the first three years of their life. Since all grown-ups walk on their heels, there is only one uniform role model that is imitated. The grown-ups were also children once. They learnt walking/marching by imitation as well. This example of the heel-walk is so consequently demonstrated and copied, that statistically it has to apply as the norm.

The realisation that the human is actually a ball-gaiter and not a heel-walker, was of such clarity and simplicity for me, that I believed that I could declare it to the whole world in one sentence. However orthopaedics and other medical practitioners didn't react accordingly.

There have certainly been reasonable orthopaedics all the time, who instead of prescribing insoles, recommended rehabilitation through strengthening exercises of the foot muscles after operations and for deformed feet. Nevertheless, the doctors could apparently never clearly distance themselves from the medical dogma of properly rolling off of the feet, in order to get to the idea that the human is genetically a forefoot-gaiter. Apparently, due to adapting the heel-walk that we learned, we all suppress the ball-gait so very much, that theoretically we're not even interested in the walking pattern of human beings any more. The human seems to be a "follower" from the first step onwards.

By the way, we learn through imitation not only in walking, but also in our language. The phase of sole imitation ends with the third year of life. The phase of imitation is a realm of consciousness that is replaced with a subsequent realm of consciousness in such a manner that it is then forgotten. Could it be that in our subconsciousness – touched by our walking behaviour – we remember how difficult it actually was for us to train our baby body to do the heel-walk? Perhaps we are scared that everything that has to do with learning would only burden us with new stress? And a further gripping question comes to me: do we perhaps have such problems developing humane school systems because of the comprehensive learning of this muscular wrongdoing in the whole body?

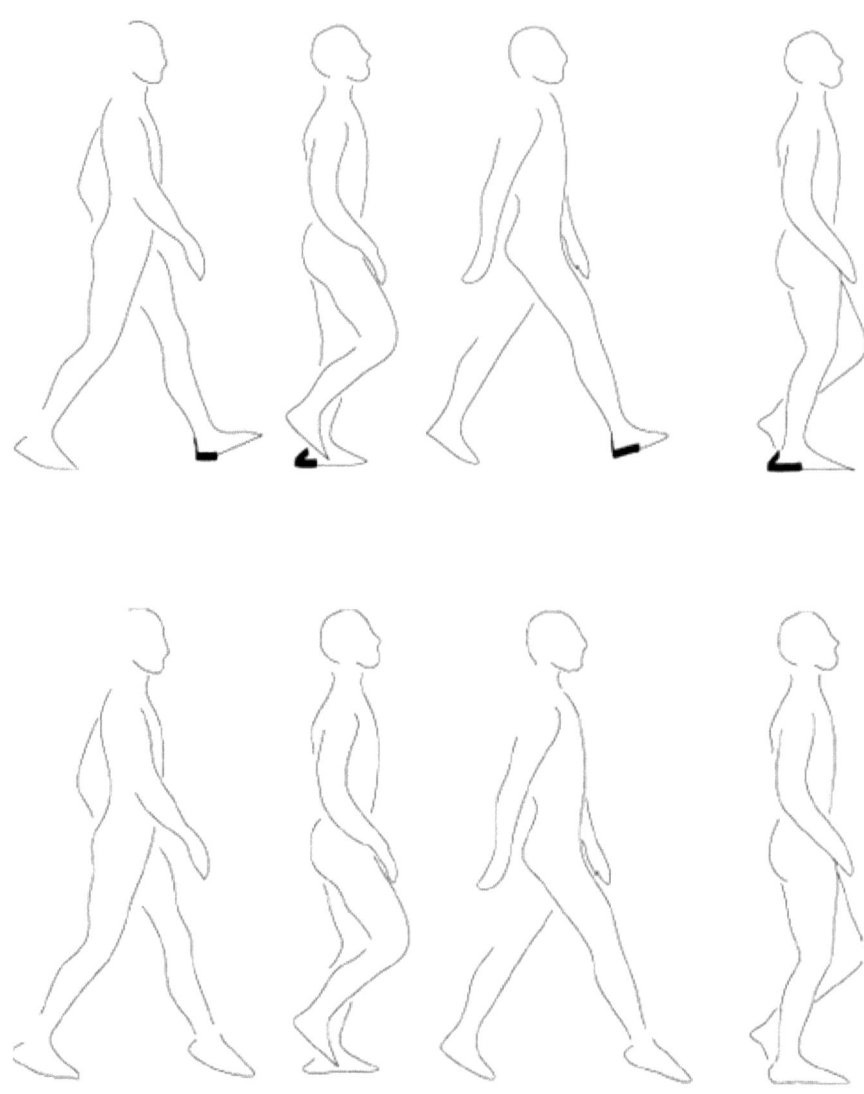

The Walking Performance of the Human

*"The true wonder isn't in
walking on water,
but on walking on the earth."*

Thich Nhat Hanh:
I plant a smile

The Platonic Soul Skills and GODO

Plato described the soul in the following three things: wanting – thinking – feeling. Goethe internalized this insight in his poem, which has become a folk-song: "I walked in the woods just for me, and looking for nothing, that was my purpose …" He allowed himself to be led for a walk by his soul.

After a thirty year long study of the Goethe inheritance in Weimar, Rudolf Steiner, the later founder of anthropology and Waldorf schools, recognised that wanting, thinking and feeling are the three activities of our soul. He explicitly called them: ACTS OF THE SOUL. Thereby the body becomes the instrument of expression of these three acts of the soul. So our walking is also an expression of it; it can be experienced in every single step.

Up until now this has only been made use of in Curative Eurhythmics. With tripartite pacing, "lifting – carrying – placing" (wanting – thinking – feeling), it has a healing effect on physical, lingual and perceptual disorders.

Stutterers express wanting – thinking – feeling at the same time. A speech knot is formed, which can be disentangled by conscious walking, that means with slowing down each of the single acts of the soul (Curative Eurhythmics).

The platonic skills of the soul are used curatively eurhythmical, solely therapeutic, or like a new mode of art based on eurhythmics. I have only met a few people who emerged as ball-gaiters from such an education. Some of the former members of the Loheland-Schule in Hessen, Germany, who have followed the anthropological principles are amongst them. Ruth Arion, the Israeli artist (1912–1988) also came into contact with this movement in her youth. She remembers having stepped the "royal gait" between 1926 and 1936. During our conversation it became clear to her that it was after her flight from the Nazis and during her work on the assembly line in the kibbutz, that she forgot the "royal gait". Many years later I was able to remind her of it again.

Every step can be grasped as a result of gestures. These gestures are, as we have experienced, an expression of the acts of our soul. Their meaning and their sequence distinguish themselves according to our way of walking, should it be as a heel-walker or as a ball-gaiter.

Resting and wanting, both of the first phases of every step, are the same with heel-walkers and ball-gaiters:

Resting

Before all movement there is rest. When we stand, we can say: **"I rest"** With this small sentence, consciously spoken or thought, we make the gesture of resting real and tangible within us. Put the book down for one or two minutes, stand up straight with your feet parallel in shoulder width, close your eyes, breathe deeply and calmly in and out whilst doing so, and think: "I rest."

Wanting

To come out of the resting position, from standing into movement, it takes an impulse of will. For this purpose we can say to ourselves: **"I want."** In this moment the heel comes off the ground. The lifting up of the foot is an expression of an implemented impulse of the soul and happens at the same time as the "I want" gesture, as the heel leaves the ground. In order to really feel this, I ask you again to put the book down and to take a few steps. Concentrate yourself on the moment when you are aware of lifting your heel at the same time as you are speaking out loud "I want".

The Japanese master Ha ku yushi said: *"The breath of the real human being is breathing with the heels."* With the GODO meditation, which I also like to call "Dynamic GODO Yoga", the lifting of the heel corresponds to the moment of beginning to breathe in. Try it out now.

Thinking

The loose, already lifted foot, the so-called free leg, traverses the room. Whereby the outer world passes us by, we push ourselves through it, just as thoughts are always passing through our head, forming anew and fading again. And becoming aware here that the soul is saying: **"I am thinking."** In doing so, the free leg hovers freely like a thought hovers over the earth.

Opinions diverge about this section of movement. The heel-walker lifts the tip of his foot up, before he steps onto the earth with his heel, whilst the ball-gaiter lets his foot hang loosely and thus meets the earth with a sense of feeling. (note from the translator: the author wrote in German *Ge(h)fuehl*, which can be translated as feeling the walk.)

What happens here requires special observation, because it is the main problem of the heel-walk.

Gait Analysis
From the chain of bones to the muscular chain

Walking on the heels = the chain of bones

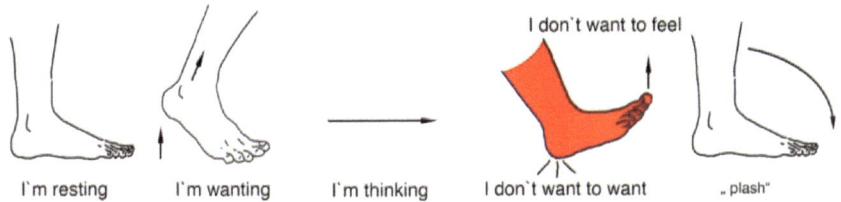

GODO = Walking on the balls of the feet = the muscular chain

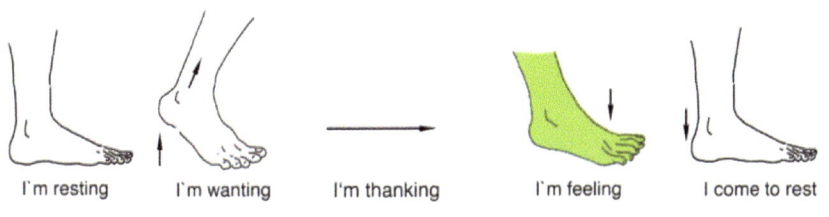

© Institut for applied human morphology   GODO - school of gait   Dr.med.Hans-Peter Greb   www.godo-impuls.com

The Gestures of the Heel-walk

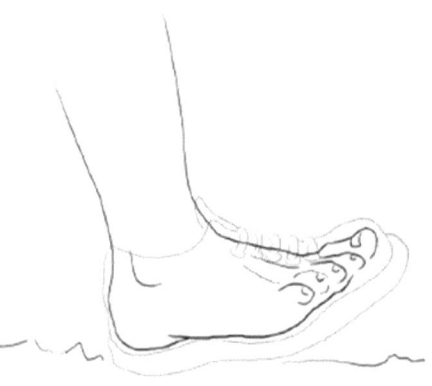

As we touch the earth with our heel first in every step, the sight of our fellow human beings who step on the earth with their heel first is so familiar to us, that we don't recognise anything conspicuous about it at first. But look again closely! It takes a special sort of concentration if you would like to capture something familiar in a new way. Take time to really do this for yourself …

Up until now such a sight was considered to be normal and natural

It's when we first analyse the heel-walk, that we understand that it not only shows a mechanical way of forward movement, but that the process itself contains a row of significant gestures with which we meet the world, and which we are responsible for in an unexpected way.

In the raised tip of the foot, the gesture of defence and the reluctance of feeling are disclosed. This expression says: "I don't want to feel, I have no trust."

It is possibile for us to express with our hands that which we unconsciously express and don't feel, with our feet. For this we can ask a completely unprepared person to reach out a hand to us. We stretch out our hand, as if we want to receive theirs, yet we pull ours back again with the gesture of defence (lifting the fingers and pushing the wrist forward).

Both are "hurt" by this paradoxical defensive gesture: the one who has caused it, and the one who is turned against.

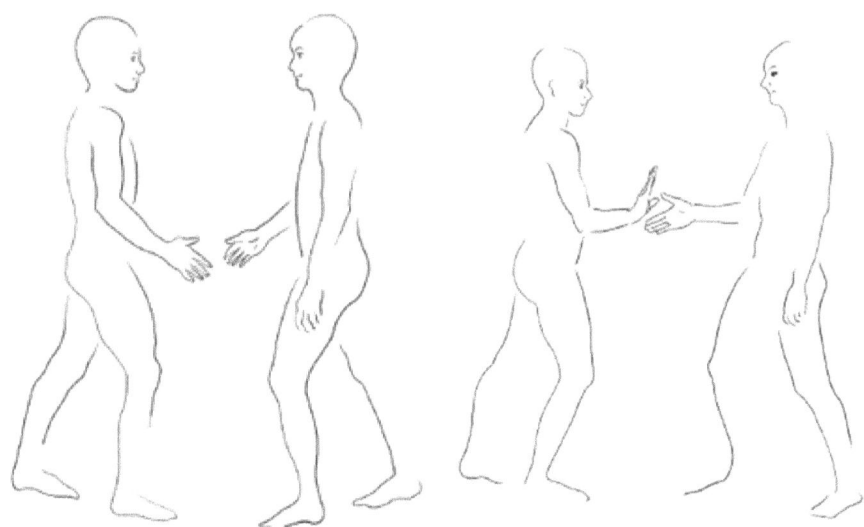

This is exactly what every heel-walker does with each step to himself, to other people and to the earth. The absurd and defensive reflection of the foot is an action done in vain. It costs us unnecessary strength and prevents the second, the intrinsic muscular action, which is needed for the completion of the venous reflux.

Does mother earth feel just as bad when we meet the ancient entity of Gaia by "forcibly walking" on the heel with the tip of the foot held-back? Could this be the reason why we move and feel like strangers on this earth, without love and awareness in doing and thinking? This gesture makes us strangers. We think, feel and act accordingly.

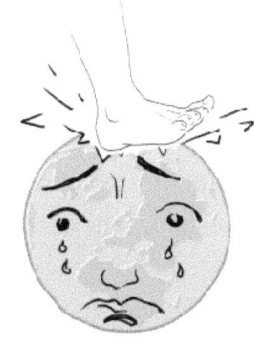

The meaning of the gesture of stamping the heel is anger and "I do not want", or "I do not want to want". As soft and fleet-footed as some individuals may walk, unrolling the feet over the heel – a certain stamping, a tremor cannot be suppressed. Soldiers marching in step can endanger a bridge with the impact of their heels. (That's why there were corresponding prohibition signs during the Second World War.) In the highest buildings in our cities, the vibration of the ground, caused by the tread of high heels, is a problem.

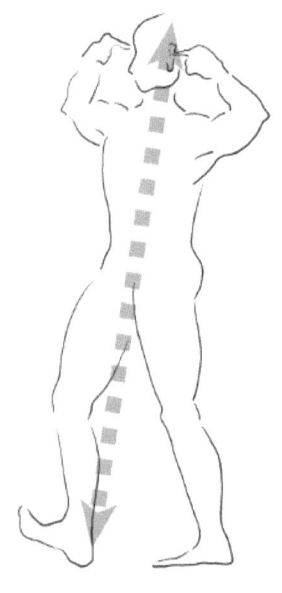

Try it for yourself: hold each of your ears closed with one finger and walk quickly in your normal fashion. Listen inside yourself. You will be able to hear a "tock-tock-tock" through your bones, which echoes from the heels up into your skull. The impact of the heels doesn't only shake the spine and the joints, and with it the muscles, but it also places unnecessary extra weight of gravity onto all of the organs. Apart from that, with every step in the heel-walk, we are continuously expressing the gestures, "I want (to start) – I don't want (feeling/wanting)". That gives a reason for a conflict of pure will. Feel into yourself when you say: "I don't want – – –." Is that not super paradox, a contradiction in itself? We land exactly where we actually wanted to go, but we are neither expressing what we want or what we feel, nor what we are willing to do. It's apparent that we cause this negating gesture actively with every step in the heel-walk, and it's logical to assume that in doing so, we install a defensive program into the brain and also into socialization.

In kinesiology a weak muscle test is caused by a defensive, denying mental attitude, and the gestures which go with it. This should give allergy researchers, amongst others, something to think about, as allergies are very often created by excessive demands.

So-called Marching on the Spot and Military Marching

Military marching is an especially distinct form of the heel-walk, in which it's walked on the heel in step. Quite the opposite holds true for the so-called marching on the spot, in which we necessarily land on the forefoot, where the arms are swung firmly and the shoulders are also moved in such a way that the whole spine performs a spiralling movement round its central axis. Try it out! For when you look very closely and feel into it, you will recognize immediately that it's about a distinct ball-striding movement. It's actually quite impossible to "march on the spot" by putting the heel down first.

As described in the chapter "Research and Insights through Observation", walking on the spot has a pronounced harmonising effect on the mind and body, meaning that the two halves of the brain are being synchronised. Kinesiologists use this, because sure tests are only possible during this state of being. Years ago, at the Congress of the Association of Kinesiologists in Kirchzarten, Germany, when I was able to explain the connection between the two this called forth great astonishment. Since then, they know that a ball-strider coming to them is already synchronised.

However, as soon as we move forwards from "marching on the spot", we involuntarily fall back into the familiar heel-walk, the real marching, which apparently causes the opposite of a harmonising effect. In marching, the arms are swung backwards and forwards in opposite directions, but the shoulders are held straight on the stiff spine. It is prevented that the middle of the body swings in a contra spiralling movement. Hip movement is also suppressed.

Towards the end of the 19th century, only Prussian officers mastered such an impeccable "goose step", that was able to impress the whole nation. The young men in the country also wanted to be like these wonderful looking Prussian cadets and officers, awakened right up to the tips of their toes. Admittedly they hadn't learnt the technical step of the parade, so that out of "normal" heel-walkers, a large army of marching soldiers ran out from the school benches. Because military marching represented an increase of the plain heel-walk, the feeling of gravity and aggression in every soldier became stronger with each impact of the heel –
unconsciously of course. The increase of their individual mass circulated collectively in the large mass of them and seemed to be carried by them. What remained unaware up until now, suddenly becomes felt through GODO.

GODO shows: **Whoever once strides, never marches again.**

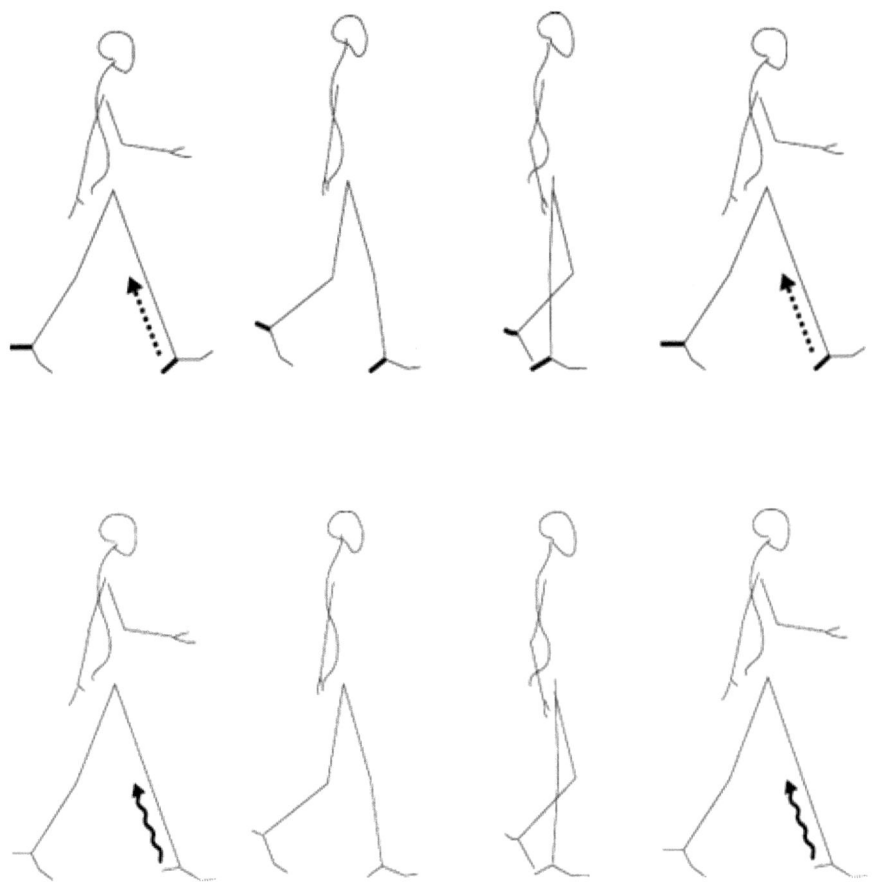

The Gestures of the Ball-gait

Feeling

*"If you don't feel it,
you will never catch it!"*

Johann Wolfgang von Goethe

The ball-gait could liberate the heel-walker from his divided nature (a chronic ambivalence) of the constant "I want – I don't want". The ball-gaiter simply refrains from not wanting. The automatic result of it is that the loose foot can softly come onto the earth with the gesture of "I feel".

After "I want", the forefoot hangs so loosely that it automatically touches the earth with the ball of the foot and the toes first. Here is a helpful exercise to prepare for this: stand with your whole weight on one leg and shake your other foot out loosely. In doing so, the foot isn't actively moved, rather it hangs down loosely from the ankle.

GODO shows: treading, we feel the softness and aliveness of the earth; in the same moment we ourselves become soft, alive and peaceful.

In English, the words "sole" and "soul" are pronounced the same. As Tucholsky once suggested, let your soul really "dangle". We only need to let our foot hang loosely, just as it was in the last moment when lifting it from the ground. You can recognize here that GODO, completely different from what you would expect, is only about letting go and not about learning a new, difficult method.

We don't lift the forefoot up in vain any more. We spare ourselves the gesticulation of suppressing feelings in this way. Instead, we say inside of ourselves: "I feel", and in doing so, touch the earth "walking fully with feeling" and lovingly, virtually footsying with the balls of the feet and the toes first, and then sinking the heel down to rest into standing.

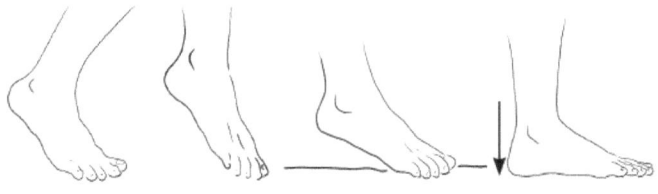

Coming to Rest

Coming to rest is sinking the heel down into the standing position. You can enjoy it very much when you have once felt it! "I come to rest." We can learn to perceive this motion and the sensations in the ankle belonging to it by carefully going backwards with dangling feet. Take a small "decelerated" step backwards from a standing position now. The foot indicates a loose hanging position, with the tip of the big toe pointing downwards and inwards, so that the primary joints of the toes are showing right-angled to the direction of movement. The foot is pronated and the arch of the foot can be distinctly observed in its concave shape in this resting position. As soon as the toes touch the ground, they send a message to the brain about the nature of the ground underneath them; our unconscious, efficient muscular balancing system stretches the spine into a vertical position and girdles the arch of the feet, so that we find our balance in a safe, flexible, stress-free manner. Practise it again and again until you feel it. It is being felt and weightless, at the same time it is effortless. Since Nena, the famous German singer, sang her song "99 Red Balloons", we all know that there is a consensus: "completely liberated" equals weightless (note from the translator – the author wrote in German *los-ge(h)-löst*, which translated means detached by walking).

Now we also understand why we cheat ourselves with high-heeled shoes. They only simulate the ball-gait, because they hinder coming to rest and the intrinsic rolling off of the feet. Indeed they make the feet virtually freeze in the pretence of "I want". Maybe the high heel is the unconscious longing for the ball-gait. We let ourselves be misled by something artificial, a prosthesis. This kind of prosthesis doesn't replace the function, rather it prevents it.

Me-Strength

Enjoy the wave of well-being coming from the striding feet emerging now in the whole body. Balance your head effortlessly on an erect spine. When you have arrived so sensitively and softly on the earth with the balls of the forefeet, the lowering of the heel into the stand begins. This lowering is a palpable way, is coming to rest, and you know, the palpable way is the aim. As heel-walkers, until now you have only been raising your forefeet up (the gesture of "I don't want to feel you") and you have fallen on the heels into your chain of bones with the posture of a hollow back,, helplessly faltering, searching for balance. Viewed as such, we, as heel-walkers, are painstakingly burdened and are very scared of falling. For this reason the heel-walker knows neither coming to rest nor real resting. Just take a look at the human world, how they are rushing and hurrying and so often suffer from trouble getting to sleep and sleeping through the night.

With GODO you slowly let the shackles of your feet go and waken up to a new experience of better straightening up in your body, your Me-strength! If you should be hesitating, bear in mind that we heel-walkers are so very much caught up in the contradiction "I want – I do not want", that it's often difficult for us to make clear decisions, even when the insight is already there.

From Thinking to Thanking

"If you muster up the fire in your heart and put it into the tantien (bladder, pelvic floor) and the centre of the feet, then the breast and diaphragm will become cool of their own accord, and you will have no shadow of speculation and thought, not any waves of thoughts and feelings." (Ha ku yushi)

If the gesture of the feet whilst doing the heel-walk is "I think", then it becomes "I thank" with the ball-gait. Because the ball-gaiter makes no reflexion (bending back) of the foot, he stays relaxed. He can thus stride through the world with an inner attitude of thankfulness, and in doing so can take in everything without being irritated by the gesture of thinking, of "reflecting". Because he has given up the reflexion, the rebellion, the gesture of "I do not want", he moves with ease and sensitivity with an undivided will – "I want". With the gift of his being, of the body. Thankful.

A hint: remember (in German *Gedenken* = go thinking); thoughts (in German *Gedanken* = go thanking). In remembering we are in the past, we think about our ancestors or our sins. When we are thinking, we tend to reach out or think back to where we are going or want to be. When we are thanking and being grateful, we are in the here and now of the perfect feeling of our body and soul. So thinking is never as satisfying as thanking.

In order that we don't misunderstand each other: retrospective remembering, whether of a personal or a historical nature, can definitely be valuable for apprehending the essence of being.

The secret success of GODO literally lies in the transition from thinking (from the reflection of the foot, reflection = thinking) to thanking. GODO shows: whoever is thinking, is still searching, but whoever is thanking, has already found. And whoever is thanking, has already received.

With GODO everyone is given the impulse to be on the beam with the progressive quintuple striding of – resting, wanting, thanking, feeling, coming to rest – to harmonically live out the skills of his soul from now on. So induced by striding, the ball-gaiter gradually blossoms into the full flowering of his being as a human, into his original, dynamic straightening up. This is the foundation of the ME who moves freely, liberated from any fear of falling (see the chapters "Fear of Falling, Ego and Superego" and "The SELF"). By striding we can achieve integration into the SELF, with an inner attitude of gratitude for life. The ball-gait releases psychic and physical strength and brings the person practising GODO into the centre of his being, the ME in the SELF. GODO shows: step for step, with deep, free breathing, the ball-gaiter experiences a rhythm of more liberated and more conscious movement – "in order to stride through life with a good feeling of self-worth", as Clemens Kuby describes the Todas, the ball-gaiting people in his book *"Unterwegs in die Nächste Dimension" (Out and about in the Next Dimension)*.

Gait and ME-development

*"There is only one temple in the world,
and that is the human body.
Nothing is more sacred than this tall
figure ..."*

Novalis

It is known that the upright walk, language and the Me consciousness distinguishes humans from the animal world. (Note from the translator: in German I is used for ME and I is everybody's original name). The development of language is connected to the erecting of the body and to the upright walk (see the chapter "Gait and Language"). And according to Steiner, the ME is the upright body posture. Psychology expresses this nowhere else so precisely.

In the following, I would like to transfer this statement onto the physical and psychological development of the child up until the third year of life. A few drawings may serve to present the individual steps of erecting for this...

The first attempts of erecting can be noticed in the lifting of the small head, which is still very wobbly and always "falls down" again. This I would like to call the unstable erecting. It corresponds to the UNSTABLE ME.

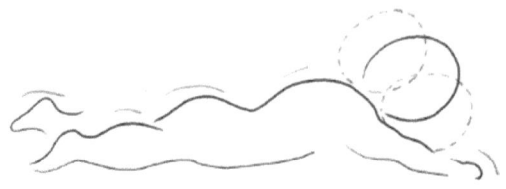

The next stage of erecting reaches perfection in the upright sitting baby, in a small Buddha. When we take a look at such a child, we notice its centerdness and its special ME-strength. Nothing really brings it to fall over – it would be more likely to roll. That's why I would like to call it the ORB-ME here. These children emit such inner strength and an undisturbed condition of ME, without being able to say the little word "me"!

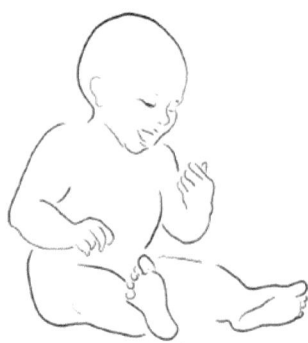

A further stage of development we come across is the child in the so-called crawling stage. In this stage of erecting you can talk of the development of the AUTOMOBILE ME (Greek: *"autós"*, German: *"selbst"*). This crawling stage is held by orthodox medical practitioners, kinesiologists and development psychologists as a crucial stage for proper physical and mental development. Attention: just because almost one hundred per cent of all children in our culture go through a crawling stage, it is not an absolute precondition for the development of a good limbic system, the so-called emotional centre. I would only like to recollect tribes such as Indians, Eskimos and Tibetans, who carry their children bundled up and stretched for up to a year. Upon setting them down for the first time, they can nonetheless start to walk and have nevertheless developed a healthy emotional world in a natural way.

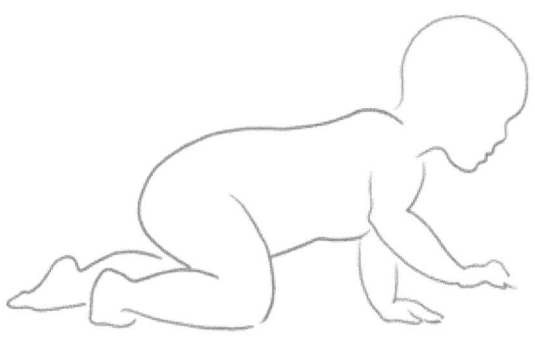

Supporting what has been said, here is a short story about research on young swallows and their learning to fly. For a long time it was held for true that young, full-fledged swallows would still flutter for a few days and learn to fly whilst hanging in the nest. In a very simple attempt, this assumption could be disproved. Three out of six little swallows coming from a clutch of eggs were put into small cardboard tubes, so that they could still be fed, but were not able to take part in the flight exercises. Not until the other three had finally flown from the nest after exercising for days on end, were the three captivated ones released. And lo and behold, without having exercised, they flew after the others! The conclusion is: when genetic maturity is reached, the function can be exercised. Accordingly, it would be better to speak of the development or the maturing of an ability in genetic specifications, than of learning them.

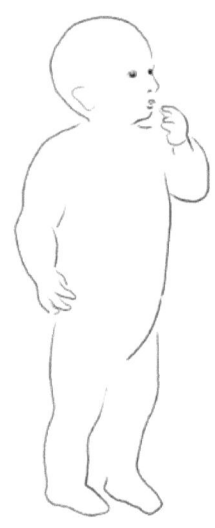

Next follows the getting upright of the whole body. We find this in the standing child. With people born by regular birth, it takes place around the time of the first year in life. The nervous system of the child is mature and permits it to stand. This standing conforms with the structural erecting and thereby with the STATIC ME. How wonderfully strong the self-consciousness of the children seem to be at this stage!

Unfortunately you frequently see parents proudly holding their children between their legs by their little hands at this stage, demonstrating upright walking. In doing so, they literally mislead them to amble in a standing foot position. Arm and leg are not moved crosswise in opposite directions, but are moved forward in the same direction. The child is being forced to learn the heel-walk and has no chance to develop its natural ball-gait. The nervous system is not mature enough for the spontaneous happening of the ball-gait.

When your child begins to stand, please play with him in the horizontal position of the preceding stage, crawling and creeping. Hold it playfully by its lower legs or by its feet for example, whilst supporting his abdomen, so that it can pick up a toy itself, which has been thrown away or has fallen.

A US-American Doctor of Chiropractic Justin Klein recommends crawling as babies for grown-ups. The newest fitness trend crawling can be found in the internet.

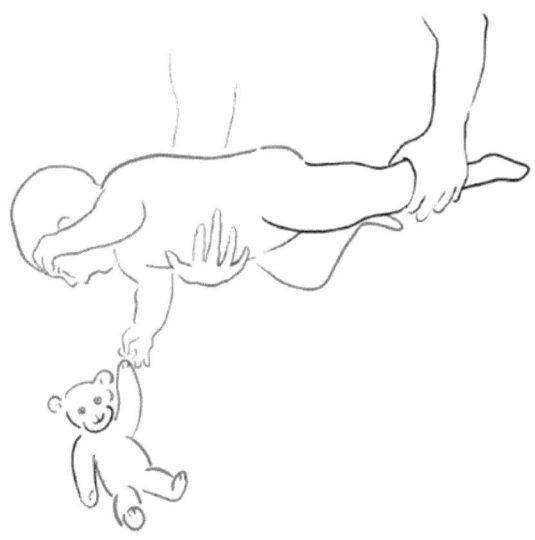

Trust in the natural development of the steps which have been genetically laid out in your child. It gains inner stability and security if it is encouraged to discover what it can do for itself. It is always more favourable for the development of movement to give more inner stability and security to children's speed of development by training the abilities of each one of the previous stages, instead of predetermining its natural development.

Now the upright forward movement, the dynamic straightening of the body posture begins. From this time on our DYNAMIC ME develops. It happens quite suddenly. With small baby steps and slightly raised little arms, we all ran off at one time without having had a practising phase beforehand. We could walk, just like the swallows could fly, because the set-up of our nerves was mature for it, and not because we had learned it beforehand. It happens simply due to our genetic structure.

We scuttled off on the balls of our feet. That demonstrated most clearly that we are actually inherently ball-gaiters.

But unfortunately, before too long we all began to learn to walk on the heels. You remember that children learn solely by imitation up until the end of the third year in their life. So we learned to imitate a walk and a pattern of movement which goes against our nature.

Parents often react to the first independent footsteps of their children by transferring their own fear of falling onto them (see also the chapter "Regular Birth, Power – Powerlessness Defiant Behaviour, Sexist Socialisation"). Which means they are scared that the child could fall or walk into something, so they incline to interfere with the first footsteps the child takes. In doing so, they disturb the spontaneous development of the movement of the small ball-gaiter in two different ways at the same time, without being aware of it. First of all their fear is transmitted onto the mind of the child: children still live fully wrapped-up in the auric emotional body of the parents; they feel fear without knowing that it isn't their own. Secondly the parents react quickly with "rescuing motions" and disrupt the children in finding their own balance. So it is being prevented that the child starts standing alone and comes to rest. This has deep effects on the last stage of our ME-development. In actual fact, in the appropriate sensitive phase, we can never develop into a perfectly achieved ME-maturity on time (see the chapter "Pregnancy, Birth and the "Sensitive Phase" ").

Fear of Falling, Ego and Superego

Using the feet as "sensitive feeling feathers", we are light-footed and balanced, just as dancers are. So with every step we carry a new, elastic and fall-safe upright body posture into the world. With the heel-walk, on the other hand, we practise a continual falling onto the heels. As a static Me, we learned to fall stepwise. The fear of falling, which accompanies us from step to step our whole life long, is something that we hardly notice. We have compensated it in a very questionable way by dividing ourselves. The Ego and the Superego is created. Balance is impaired by the reflective conduct of the feet in the heel-walk. This balance is part of the static erecting, and belongs to the static Me. And the already perfected harmony of the Me-maturity of a one-year-old standing child subsequently becomes insecure. Yes, you could say that after this, each one of us stalks through the world as an unsure one-year-old Me.

To compensate for this insecurity caused by the fear of falling, the child searches for dependency and support by imagining two psychosocial psychological spaces for itself, which are an illusion:

1. By saying: "I am strong like Superman, I feel no pain", it creates the ego. In doing so, it practises lying about itself, as it isn't as big and strong as Superman or as Dad yet, and humiliation and pain are suppressed. Fantasies of being omnipotent are being created here, which is the ego. Now we know how and why and when your ego came into being. For the first time it's now clear what the ego actually is, from which – without this knowledge – we try to rid ourselves of in vain. Now we can really define the source of it. Not being aware of of the above, caused that English speaking scientists use the expression ego when I or me is actually meant.

2. As Superego it says about itself: "like this I behave well, exactly like Mum and Dad." Here we are all entering some identification which alienates us from ourselves for as long as we can't figure it out, and that makes us have a bad conscious under the surface all the time. (Note from the translator: bad conscious in German = *schlechtes Ge(h)wissen* = we have a bad knowledge of walking.)

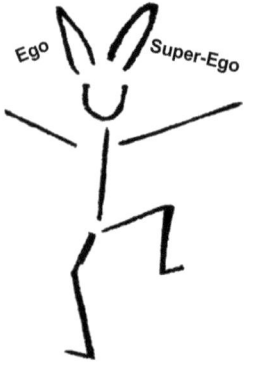

Out of the wonderful static Me has now become a sort of a matchstick man Me in danger of falling, with two psychic bubbles of lies (Ego and Superego), which I describe here as large dog's-ears. Instead of that, out of what was the relatively healthy child up until the static Me, could have become a gloriously flexible human being with an undivided, undisrupted, dynamic Me.

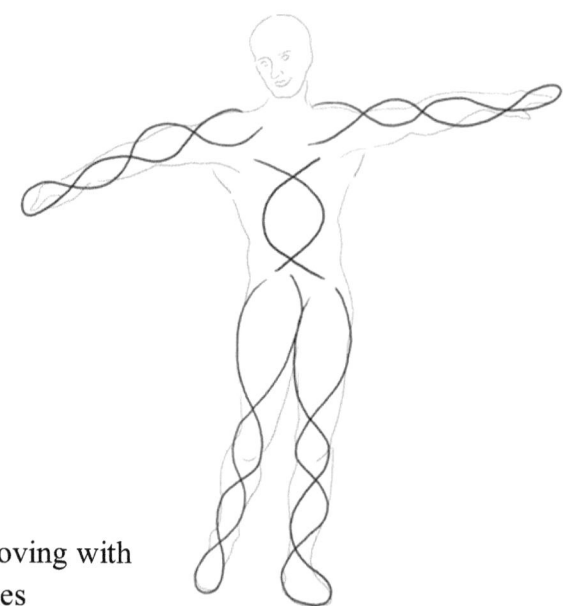

A human being moving with the chain of muscles

There is at least one famous example in the world for such a development: Vaslaw Nijinsky, the great, yes, probably the greatest dancer, who never took part in the conditioning of the heel-walk. Up until the tenth year of his life, and so up until the discovery of his dancing talent, he was a rural socialized ball-gaiter. Unfortunately, in being so, he didn't know that he was different from almost all other people – also from other ballet dancers, who almost exclusively perform in the forefoot emphasised dance, but when they leave the stage and go home, fall into the heel-walk. They didn't know, and still don't know, that they are actually ball-gaiters. Nijinsky, who didn't know that his ball-gait is the true nature of all people, is completely different. It went so far that he was the only choreographer of his time who created a heel-walk-choreography. That was the beginning of his madness. The overall corruption, represented in learning the heel-walk, did reach him at a late stage in his life. He received fanatical applause on all stages when performing and he became a box-office success, yet he soon frightened his manager by insisting to offer his performances to the people for free, on which they deemed him to be insane. Because, as a person who had not imitated the self-worth-devastating heel-walk, his self-love wasn't impaired, so almost like Jesus, he loved people just as much as he loved himself and his art. And he didn't want to sell his outstanding example, but wanted to give it to them all for free. None of his managers could understand such a consequent social attitude. Wouldn't it be wonderful if we all were so socially developed?

This story shows in a special way that the completed development of the ME doesn't only allow the body to grow into perfection, it also entails a very high psychosocial integration. Even though Vaslaw Nijinsky grew up as a child of nature and as a ball-gaiter outside of the area of cultural hustle and bustle, he was able to easily integrate himself into the "big world", without even corrupting his social soul. Has he not been far ahead of us heel-walkers? In his autobiographic book *"The Clown of God"*, he describes himself and the people around him in the increasingly unbearable division between his authenticity and their artificiality. Unfortunately he didn't know anything about GODO.

The SELF

At this point I would like to say something about the SELF. There seems to be no real clarity prevailing about what it really is. On the one hand we are all trying to recognize it, indeed a lot of people even pay a lot for so-called self-awareness seminars and workshops; on the other hand we swear on the SELFLESSNESS as being an especially desirable condition. What you have to buy for yourself, you most likely don't have. And as there are so many people who are looking for it, it's rather interesting to find out where we may have lost it or where we could have missed the path to ourselves.

According to GODO, I would like to offer you the following thoughts here: **Only a fully developed ME is capable of experiencing integration into the SELF!** That means: when a child has ended the third year as a ball-gaiter instead of as a heel-walker, it is naturally matured. It has fulfilled its genetic plan in such a way that it is able to experience what we can call "the integration of the ME into the SELF". It feels properly matured, harmonic and in balance, and can now open itself to the world, to the whole, and to the SELF.

In turn, we must consequently accept that a human being with the usual conditioning of a heel-walker can hardly feel fully integrated into this world. For the integration into the SELF also happens during a sensitive stage (see the chapter "Pregnancy, Birth and the "Sensitive Phase" "), just between the third and the fifth year of life. Only during this sensitive stage can we experience the development of the "sense for the SELF". The sense of the SELF, as such, is not yet known. Do we perhaps have the feeling of having been driven out of paradise so easily due to this?

Circulation, Emotional Body and Gender Emancipation

The topics of gender emancipation, emotional bodies and the return of the venous blood to the heart are illuminated anew with GODO and brought into a context, which hasn't ever been seen so clearly before.

Under emancipation we broadly understand the release from a state of dependency. With all that has been previously mentioned, you can imagine that a lot of dependencies within our bodies must have resulted from the wrong use of the feet. In this special case, which we speak about here, the blood circulation, the organ of the emotional body e.g. the feelings and sensations is impaired by the wrong use of the foot because the heel-walk doesn't sufficiently support the venous reflux towards the heart. How is that to be understood?

The circulation exists mostly of the heart, the arteries, the capillary tubes and the veins. It is a self-contained system, which actively pumps the oxygen-saturated blood in the body by muscular contraction of the arteries, from which it passively flows back through the veins to the heart. Thus there is no thrust from the heart for the flow of blood going back, and the veins don't have any muscular tissues, like the arteries do. Nevertheless, the blood in the veins must flow straight up the body against the pull of gravity.

To the question in the medical exam, of how the blood is brought back to the heart, a significant part of the answer must be: "by the pumping of the calf muscle." Moving the feet has an active impact on our circulation. Everyone knows that movement leads to better circulation, better health and also better moods.

Most fitness devices train bending and stretching functions particularly well. An economically flowing motion in a closed muscular system (body/circulation) always describes a counter spiralling movement though. This consists of the harmonic cooperation of bending and stretching muscle power (flexors and extensors), plus rotating movements round the axis of the bones at the same time, performed by muscles rotating inwards and muscles rotating outwards (pronators and supinators).

This holistic way of thinking in synergistic muscular functions is known to physiotherapists as "complex movements". Neuromuscular interaction is thereby practised with combined functional movements, in order to connect the synaptic functions (nerve transfers) again to the natural motional pattern. With stroke-patients, e.g. bringing the food to the mouth is practised. According to GODO, the terms "muscle pump of the calf", "self-contained system", "synergistic muscular functions" and "complex movements" don't permit the term "closed system in the chain of muscles" to appear in its holistic approach.

The two different types of circulations (veins/arteries) were allocated a feminine and a masculine quality by the traditional Chinese in their Yin/Yang manner of thinking. The heart can be seen as the ideal three-dimensional embodiment of the Yin/Yang-symbol, which is familiar to everyone by now. According to this principle, our emotional body consists of a feminine, Yin part (the venous system) and a masculine, Yang part (the arterial system). One can conclude from this that a well-functioning circulation creates a harmonic ratio of feminine and masculine energies within us. We all know how certain emotions can involuntarily and expressively be felt as changes in the circulation. The cardiovascular system reacts the same way in men as in women with blushing, e.g. with shame, or by becoming pale with shock, in the beating of the heart, or in having butterflies in the stomach. Emotional agitation expresses itself through reactions in the circulation by being seen and felt. When the blood pressure is too low or too high, it also affects our mood. The subject of many proverbs and songs are hearts, as we perceive our feelings in the heart.

As said, the huge calf-muscles become pumps for the blood. They help to bring back the venous blood to the heart, against the pull of gravity. In order to do that effectively, it takes the right sequences of movement in the feet. The two rolling movements of "I want" (extrinsic) at the start of the motion and the "I come to rest" (intrinsic) at the end of each step, set a double muscular pump in motion. The one contraction brings us forwards, the other serves to ensure the static erecting. Together both cause not only a quantitatively intensifying back-flow, but are also qualitatively harmonising and thus relieving to some extent.

Summarised once again: because the muscular pumps are refined double and treble with GODO, venous blood doesn't accumulate in the legs as it does with the heel-walk. The heel-walker always suffers from the consequences of only one simple pump of the muscle per step, which is activated with "I want". "I want" uses the extrinsic muscles. A second pumping action occurs only with the ball-gait from the setting down of the forefoot and the following intrinsic lowering with the coming-to-rest motion. With the heel-walk, with landing directly on the heel, the second muscular pumping action (intrinsic) never occurs. Walking on the heels, we are thus suppressing one of both of the possible muscular pumping actions, and in doing so we especially weaken the venous part of our circulation. The wrong use of the muscles doing the heel-walk causes a state of dependency in the venous blood flow, the feminine part of the emotional body. This is why women tend to compensate this by moving around more than men, especially in doing various chores in the household.

This means that in all heel-walkers, in men as well as in women, the feminine emotional harmony is depleted or weakened. The suppressed femininity reacts either with resignation or with an ever increasing urge for emancipation. On top of that, the arterial, the masculine part of our circulation (emotional body) is only positively strengthened in its function by the straightening up of the body posture, because then the blood gravitates downwards into the largest part of the body. The arterial, oxygen saturated, light red blood is actively pumped downwards within the erected body by the muscle power of the heart and by the muscle-coated arteries and is supported by the hydrostatic falling direction. Arterially overdriven to such an extent, men especially tend to neglect and suppress their feminine emotionality. This gives the masculine part in us such an advantage, that from an overall societal standpoint, men as well as women tend towards machismo. Does the world not suffer right now from an exaggeration of complex masculine feelings and from a common deficiency of sensitive feminine drive?

By means of GODO, we save our circulation from this one-sided burden. With the help of the harmonic double muscular pump and from that the chain-like ascending and descending, rippling movement of all the other muscles in the whole body, we acquire emancipation in ourselves in a special way. The masculine and feminine energies find their balance on the level of our circulation/emotional body. If individual harmony rules on the inside, then we can expect that it's transmitted all on its own to the outside, into society.

It turned out that e.g. in Germany thirty to fifty per cent of all marriage vows were given in conjunction with a dance. *"Touched a thousand times, a thousand times nothing happened"*, and suddenly in dancing, with the right use of our feet and our muscle chains, eyes begin to shine, and hearts begin to open for each other – *"and it made "zoom""* (Klaus Lage, a German singer). What happened? The circulation of masculine and feminine energies become harmonised in each and every dancer. Everyone loves themselves much better so, and can, as the motto goes, *"love your neighbour as yourself"*, love the other better.

I would like to briefly point out C.G. Jung's Animus/Anima concept. According to it, the psychological state of suffering in men and women depends upon a lack of fulfilment of the respective parts of the soul in the opposite-gender. With GODO, the origin of this lack is at long last comprehensible on a physical level and very precisely corrigible with the most simple self-initiative. But as always, whichever way we turn, many roads lead to the same destination.

A good example is the journalist Franz Alt. Due to a midlife crisis, which significantly expressed itself as heart arrhythmia in the central organ of the emotional body, Franz Alt found his way to dream analysis after C.G. Jung, and also felt deeply drawn to Jesus. Later he writes about it in his book *"Jesus – the first new man"*:

"The source, out of which I scoop, is Jesus. I got to know Jesus as an anima-integrated man. The masculine one-sidedness of understanding, which prevails up until today in us men (partly in women too), separates, suppresses, denies and demonises everything feminine, and accounts for the real madness of our times."

Jesus' perfected ME-consciousness is equivalent to the resurrection in flesh, meaning that, Jesus is also a symbol for the successfully perfected, dynamic manner of uprighting. I can only imagine this in a ball-gaiter …

As a brochure from 1996 from the DAK (*Deutsche Angestellten Krankenkasse* = German health insurance for employees) about education on veins disclosed, already more than 20 million people in Germany suffered from vein diseases at that time. 9 million of those became patients per calendar quarter. We may presume that most of these sufferers could have liberated themselves from this suffering by healing themselves with the ball-gait – or would not even have become ill.

By walking the GODO way we liberate our circulation from lopsided stress. Emancipation through GODOing liberates everyone emotionally. With the help of the harmonised double muscle pump (intrinsic extrinsic), the muscle chain functions without disrupture. If harmony reins within, we can expect that it projects itself into the outward sphere and into society, healing the social realm.

Whoever is balanced on the inside, can meet the other gender more easily and consciously. In this way social relationships can be continuously improved on the outside, being seen as a mirror of the relationships of the inner world of each and every self-responsible individual.

GODO shows: The ball-gait lessens the battle between the sexes.

Research and Insights through Observation

Biomechanists from the physical education college in Cologne, Germany, developed with Prof. Baumann an ideal curve of printed images that a walking foot should be making on the earth. They examined different top athletes for this, in order to be able to determine which manner of using the foot (with the emphasis on the ball of the foot, the side or the heel) empowered them to achieve higher performance. None of these sportsmen reached the ideal curve. Also with people who are untrained, who walk as is usual, on the heels, the calculated picture was never achieved. Through striding in GODO however, this curve can be reached at any time.

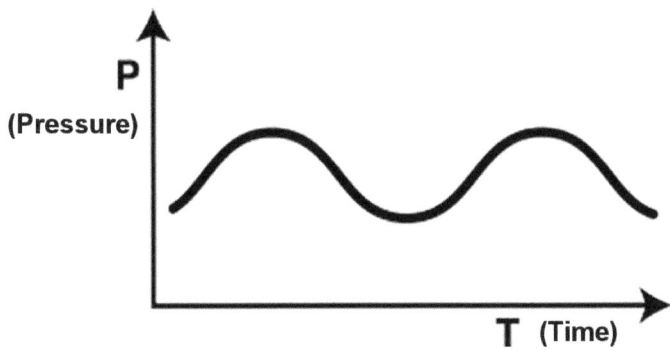

Thirty years ago in the Institute for Biomechanics in Cologne, Germany, the step on the heel was already calculated with an average of 50 kilograms. This means that with every step on the heel we strain our skeleton with this unnecessary weight. Calculate this please: 100 steps of 50 kilograms gives 5 tons. This approximately represents the weight of two Porsche cars. As a heel-walker you kick the earth on the one hand and you also kick yourself as a counter-blow in the backside. An eighty-year-old has covered around about the distance of 120000 kilometres in the course of his life, which is three times around the earth. This coincidentally represents the weight of the pyramid of Giza.

Under the supervision of Prof. G. Schumpe, atomic scientist, doctor and the former manager of biomechanics at the orthopaedic university clinic on the Venus Berg in Bonn, research of walking motions took place with special consideration on the GODO "theories" in parenthesis, because it is indeed a fact and not a theory. With the help of the ultrasonic-topographic system developed by him, he is able to allow three-dimensional motion pictures to appear on the monitor. With this, it was possible to make very precise statements about the strain on the joints and the strength needed in practising the different motions of walking. One thing became clear in this pictural method: in the forefoot walk, the swing of the head, depending on the step, in the vertical as well as in the horizontal, was on the average over fifty per cent less than with the heel-walk. The GODO motion picture is more harmonic and in any case also less strenuous on the joints. Since then, this discovery has been researched further in the orthopaedic practice of Dr med. Rainer Lueders (www.medizin-24.de), in cooperation with the sport laboratory of Thomas Stehle (www.fitexpert.de) and taught to patients and athletes.

Patients who suffer from a birth-traumatic impairment of the pyramidal tracts provide us with a different perspective on GO-DO. (The motor neurons are also called the pyramidal tracts. They conduct conscious decisions of motion from the pyramid-shaped cells in the motoric cerebral cortex into the limbs.) The still intact, partially functioning motor neurons of these patients are shown, amongst other things, by a splay foot position, which is proved to be the basic program of our actual walking movement. Learning to stand on the heel is a later development, which the pyramidal tracts of these patients are no longer capable of.

Third Scientific Proof:

It is known that in the case of paraplegia, the neural pathways underneath the injury remain intact. Commands of movement from the brain stop at the injury and don't reach below it any more. In an experiment with a paralysed patient, something very surprising took place. Through the stimulation of the peripheral nerves with electrodes, it was possible to create a sequence of movement as in walking. The test person was disappointed, because his feet didn't function as expected from the heel-walk, he was now using the forefeet to walk. Only for those used to the heel-walk, was the gait "wrong". The chain of muscles of the genetic program at the bottom of the body couldn't receive orders from the head at the top. Therewith it is proved that the heel-walk is a program from the head and an interference in our nature as a ball-gaiter.

In my long-standing practice, I could determine that so very many symptoms disappear when the patient practices GODO. As incredible as it may sound: some **asthmatic people** were able to heal from their attacks with the information alone, that the human is, genetically seen, a ball-gaiter, by immediately taking a few slow conscious GODO steps when an attack started. In doing so their breathing becomes free again (see also the chapter "The Miraculous Healing of an Eight-year-old Boy").

The German Motopedic Dr. phil. Jutta Schulke-Vandre has found out, independent of GODO, that repeated experiments in going backwards make it possible that the asthma attacks of her patients become more seldom and strongly diminish. In going backwards we are all ball-gaiters. She got especially good results by making her patients go down the stairs backwards as often as possible.

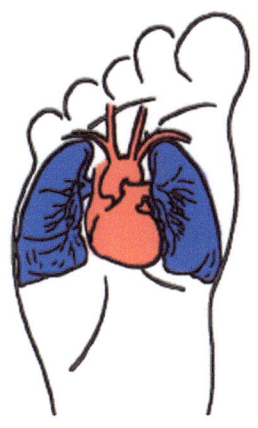

I would like to point out the well-known technique of foot reflexology at this point, and remind you that the zones for the rhythmical organs, the lungs and the heart, lie in the area of the balls of the feet. They are properly stimulated in the ball-gait, as well as by dancing. (The first four editions of this book in German had the title *"GODO – Walking with the Heart"*!)

Whoever suffers with acute **sciatica** and are not able to take another step on the heel, are often helped with the information to allow the foot to be loose and to bring the gaiting leg forwards. With the forefoot lifted upwards, the muscles on the back of the leg are stretched and the sciatic nerve is squeezed (drawing on the right). If, in contrast, you walk backwards, with the foot loose as in dancing, the painful poor posture goes (drawing). Besides, more and more orthopaedics now recommend walking backwards for complaints in the hip, knee and lumbar vertebrae.

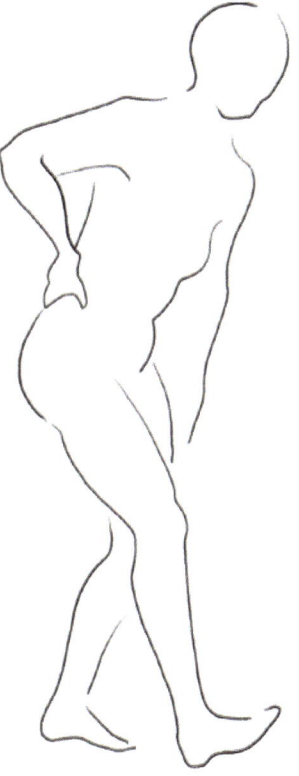

Here are some examples of the natural and instinctive transition to the ball-gait:

Perhaps the reader knows that very many Indians live in Africa. During a stay in Nairobi, I came across the Indian Odissi-dance for the first time. In this ancient art of dancing, the complete Indian mythology is represented with the hands in mudra positions. I was at training several times and could observe that the dancers walked several steps on the balls of the feet after coming from the stage, as their feet are used like small, expressive drums in dancing, pounding with the heels, coming from a ball-gait position, similar to the flamenco dance. In answer to my question, they explained to me that they did this to loosen the often painfully overworked joints of their feet. Due to their dancing technique, these dancers were very strongly sensitized in the ankles and heels, and had therefore become used to leaving the stage in the ball-gait. After a few steps however, they fell back into their day-to-day movement, the heel-walk, which dominates over the whole world. I took a few dancers aside and showed them GODO. The result was wonderful: the dancers who had become familiar with GODO retained the ball-gait as their daily movement. They recognised that they could make their joints more resistant with this. A real process of becoming conscious had taken place for them.

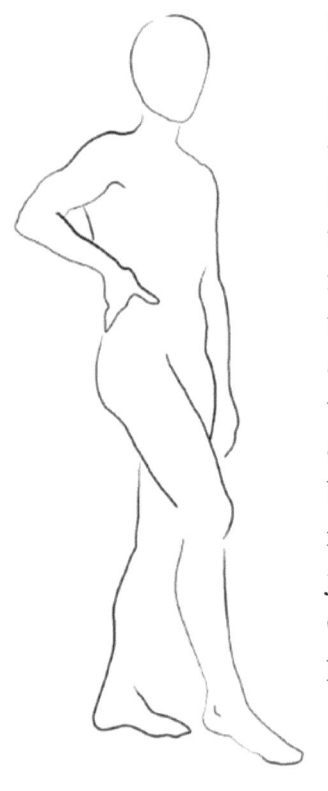

Fourth Scientific Proof:

In 1986 I followed the request of a friend to go to San Diego. He had gained experience for himself with the newest Russian biofeedback machines there, which Dr. Frank Sullyvan used in his Institute for the Synchronisation of Hemispheres (the synchronization of electrical processes in both parts of the cerebrum). This friend already knew about the hypothesis of GODO for a number of years. As he was a very strong and successful "masculine" man, he couldn't overcome himself to be seen in the ball-gait on the street. Yet after he had one of Dr Sullyvan's biofeedback treatments behind him, he experienced how he automatically walked out of the test chamber in the ball-gait, and could playfully walk easy in GODO for a whole day long. I travelled there with a group of eight German doctors, and we were able to observe that most of the test persons, who had a successful synchronisation of both halves of the brain, walked involuntarily for some minutes on the balls of the feet. Here it could be proved, that a thorough harmonising of the nervous system spontaneously brought about the ball-gait.

Muscle-tests, as in kinesiology, require a basic fundamental synchronisation of the hemispheres. Non-synchronised patients are difficult to test. As the Austrian non-medical practitioner Sissi Karz found out, a short-term synchronisation of the hemispheres in very sick patients can however be reached by "marching" the test-person on the spot for five minutes. With this exercise, you can only walk on the balls of the feet. It can therefore be assumed that we owe the synchronisation of the hemispheres to the special sequence of motion in the ball-gait.

You can have such a test kinesiologically proved for yourself at any time: if you take twenty steps in the heel-walk, you will find that you are tested to be weak.

The newest American research on the treatment of depression has revealed that intensively walking stairs, which is anyway only possible in the ball-gait, shows the best results.

If Tai-Chi in the old Yang-style is done on the balls of the feet, it mobilises the life energy force especially well. Unfortunately this is borne in mind far too seldom. The same goes for the wonderful Qigong exercises.

Time and again it's appeared evident that with PNF (Proprioceptive Neuromuscular Facilitation), the client treated on the table takes several steps on the forefoot after standing up, mostly without being aware of it himself. Even the practitioners first noticed it after we made them aware of it. What happened here? The treatment, made up out of a combination of contact stimulus and complex motions with adapted resistance, which is evoked by the practitioner on the client, activates patterns of inborn motion in the central brain.

"This overflow of activity in other sections of the body is called irradiation. One also speaks of a targeted, typical walk irradiation, as the entire motional pattern of walking is stored in the central nervous system after the sensomotorical development as a child."
(http://de.wikipedia.org/wiki/Propriozeptive_Neuromuskuläre_Fazilitation)
Here I point out the fact that the motional patterns of walking are still persistent and have not undergone an evolutionary genetic change by the general imitation of the heel-walk.

What about Indigenous People?

The ball-gait can still be found with some of the indigenous people today: whilst I – as a two-metre-man – followed the Pygmies deeply bent over on their foot-width paths through the jungle, I could observe that they removed all of the little sticks from the path with a small movement of the tip of the foot, then tentatively set down their feet on the forefoot – and under this condition they are consequently ball-gaiters. This corresponds in a way with the stalking of hunters, should it mostly be to prevent the cracking of sticks.

The author Christopher McDougall reports in his famous book *"Born to Run – A Forgotten Nation and the secret of the best and happiest Runners in the world"* about the unbelievable running performance of the Tarahumara. They run quite a few marathon stretches one after the other barefoot through the Mexican wilderness in the ball-run, or in quite old-fashioned non-damped, flat, cheap sport shoes. Were the Tarahumaras formerly ball-gaiters?

With the American Indians, the basic step with which they always dance their Powwows, is initially with a light touch upon the earth with the tip of the foot, and then a ball-emphasised step. Seen from the GODO perspective, it looks as if they wanted to deliberately point out to the ball-gait with this dance. In doing so, the modern-day American Indian isn't aware of the meaning of this. Although for example from Carlos Castaneda's description of the "Walk of Power" in *"The Journey to Ixtlan",* it has become known that the ball-emphasised exercise of the intensive "on-the-spot-pattering" makes quick motion possible, which takes a person unhurt and above all very quickly through impassable terrain, even in complete darkness.

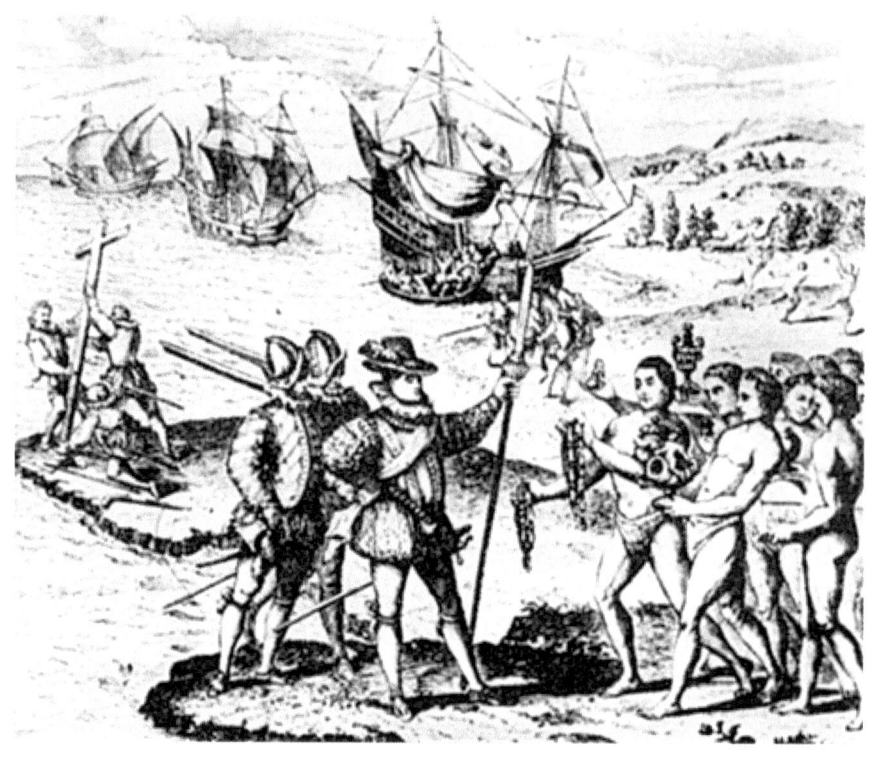

With Aborigines, who are by now heel-walkers, there is the condition of not touching the earth with the heels whilst performing sacred initiation rites.

Clemens Kuby reports in his book *"Unterwegs in die nächste Dimension" (On the Way into the next Dimension)* about the Todas, a small southern Indian tribe of not even one thousand people. As vegetarians, they have formed a symbiotic relationship with wild buffaloes, by the buffaloes giving them their milk. They know no fear, they have no religion and they feel rich. They walk *"barefoot on the fields in their surrounding area, as they don't want to step with shoes on the food of their brothers and sisters"*. They walk elegantly, quickly and *"carry the stretched foot quite close to the ground and place it down on the ground from the ball to the heel. In doing so, they are more able to feel where they tread. And they bend everything gently to the side that stands tall on the ground before they put their weight down. If an animal is on the path that they don't notice in time, they feel it with their toes and are able to pull the foot back or to step over it, because their weight is still on the other foot behind."*

We, from the so-called civilised tribes, only spontaneously react on very uneven ground with the ball-gait. As already mentioned, our feet have "gone to sleep" with progressive secondariness on evened ground. Nevertheless, the ball-emphasised use of the feet is alive in us all in ballet, in dancing, in sprinting, in boxing, in climbing stairs and in stalking. These are especially dynamic movements. We also express our joy by lifting ourselves up onto the balls of the feet. When a child readily wants to come along, it tripples with excitement.

In contrast, the heel-walk is rather harder, firmer, stiffer and more robot-like. Strictly speaking, we walk on our heel bones like on crutches. Stepping assertively on the heels, we then want to demonstrate our anger, or we are wildly determined against something. The worst is the highly developed heel-walk in marching. The experience we make as heel-walkers makes us fear the "hard impact" with the heels so much, that we don't expect anything good from smooth, hard ground. Here is a small insight: as a practising GODO, it's extremely great fun to meet the highly polished stone grounds in churches and banks, or even just the even, hard road surface.

Evolution

Reptilian Brain and the Heel Bone

The form of the human heel bone also deserves special consideration, as apart from us, we only find a heel bone of the same shape in the crocodile. That's evolutionary and genetically a completely overlooked fact. At the basis of the uprighting of our body posture, a 500 million year old crocodile gene has ironically taken shape and made our evolutionary relation to reptiles blatantly obvious.

As Darwin proved our relation to the apes, it was a shock for the human self-image. The Vatican, significantly enough, first recognised the theory of evolution at the end of 1996. Today we know that humans and chimpanzees have identical genes to almost ninety-nine per cent.

How much truth lies in the comparison of humans to the brainless crocodile, which only has the brain stem and the olfactory brain at its disposal? The main task of the brain stem restricts itself to the management of survival programs: eating, drinking, reproduction, fighting, fleeing and sleeping or the playing dead reflex. This reptilian brain, the oldest evolutionary part of the brain, the brain stem, is still placed at the base of our brain today. It has the same functions in us as it does in the crocodile. As described in the following, it becomes irritated by the heel-walk, and is held in a stressed condition with it.

The crocodile uses its heel bone in the heel-walk, crawling horizontally. Only in mating does it sometimes become upright. Then it only *stands* – and doesn't walk! For us humans, the heel bone usually serves us as a solid stand. It is our "standing-bone".

In this context I would like to remind you again of the FOOT REFLEX ZONES, as the zones for the testicles and the ovaries just happen to lie in the middle of the heels. In abusing the heels by walking on them, we irritate the sexual organs with each and every step (50 kilograms). The common well-versed person already suspects it: the heel-walker "walks on his own balls". Apart from that, we compress the joints (hips and lower back) with the recoil in such a way that the pelvic organs (intestines and reproductive organs) are often insufficiently and irregularly supplied with blood and innervation. This leads to a counterproductive simultaneity of stimulation and blockage in the sexual sphere (note from the translator: in German this is *Geschlechts-Bereich*. The author wrote *Ge(h)schlechts-Bereich*, which literally translated means "go-badly-area".) Is there possibly an explanation here for the so commonly impaired relationship to our sexuality and to our whole lower body? (Note from the translator: impaired in German is *gestört*. The author writes *ge(h)stört*, which emphasises the connection with walking, *gehen* in German.)

In two fully different ways, the heel-walk has on the one hand, an effect on our motional pattern and thus on our gestural appearance in the world, and on the other hand on our inner perceptions of the world. The latter relates to the very probable effect on our reptilian brain (brain stem and olfactory brain) caused by the impact of the heel strike. This part of the brain is also called the brain stem and lies in the spinal canal in the passage of the cervical spine into the head, where we are particularly exposed to every superfluous and unphysiological burden in an unprotected way ("hard knocks or setbacks").

The "I want – I don't want" gesture of indecision towards the earth creates a stagnant wave of ambivalence in the heel-walker-psyche. In addition, a constant underlying irritation of the brain stem is produced, driven this time from the command centre. The organisation of the relations between the brain stem and the brain, following the irritation, is particularly expressed in social behaviour, which seems to have stood still on a reptilian level. This is namely the belief of orgasm-fixated sex, excessive eating and drinking, as well as the fight and flight mechanisms apparently as the most significant and fully legitimate basic principles for survival. Our apology for that is self-preservation. An interesting tantric approach in trying to cope with the conflict can be found in Barry Long's book *"Nur die Angst stirbt" (Only the Fear Dies)*.

The irritated brain stem, along with its mechanically working survival program, responds so strongly in stress, that a child can be like a fury, almost like a wild animal. Such irritated children are gruff and agitated. They take over everything or push everything away, they even lash out for no reason. This causes unknowing parents to react repeatedly with most rigorous training measures. However this only makes the child either become broken, or his resistance becomes stronger, and then you wonder about the reason why he "runs completely wild". The causes for food, drink and sex addictions, as well as aggressiveness and nervousness in grown-ups in today's world can be found here.

You can assume that that which we call "upbringing" really only is a – seemingly necessary – reaction, with which we are trying to encounter the excessive impulses coming from irritations of the brain stem, which has been conditioned by the heel-walk and the fear of falling. That would mean that the brain learns via upbringing to engage in coping with these irritations, so that we can survive with them. In reality, as its controller and director, the brain becomes the slave of the brain stem. And as Albert Einstein assumed, maybe we only use ten per cent of our brain in this way?! Do we perhaps find it so difficult to behave less reactively because of that? This way we are probably creating the environment which determines our existence. Or which holds it in unnecessary limitations of taboos, morals and control?

Can it reconcile us a little to finally know now that we can ascribe the majority of our impossible behaviour to the fact that with the misuse of the heel bone, we bring ourselves down to the level of the crocodile, and that the simple transition from a heel-walker to a ball-gaiter could liberate us from this five million years ongoing self torment? **GODO shows: the ball-gait also liberates us from aggression.**

Gait and Language

In the French and the English language, which have strong Latin roots, we call the joint, as well as the pronunciation, *"articulation"*.

With the third year of life, ninety-five per cent of the organic growth of our brain is completed. By walking and talking we become functioning people. But now you should know that walking and talking use the same neural pathways, the motor neurons, which can also be called pyramidal tracts. On the one hand they are in charge of deliberate decisions and bring them to be expressed through motion; on the other hand they are a lesser known sensory organ, namely the sensory organ for the correct use of language, which can be betrayed by talking habits or bent by dialects. Walking and talking and the so-called conscious control of the breath are developed parallel to each other. The physical stress, caused by learning the heel-walk and walking life-long in this "neurotic movement", is inevitably (in the truest sense of the word) strengthened by the psychic stress caused in every step by the repetition of the contradictory gesture (I want – I don't want). (Note from the translator: in German, inevitable is *zwangslaeufig*, which literally translated means forced walking). The pyramidal tracts, the motor neurons and this lesser known sensory organ are put heavily under pressure by the heel-walk. We don't directly notice it, because we all have the same defect that is practised in "chattering", small talk and shouting wildly at each other. But if we take a look at the man-made conditions of our world, then we can easily explain many states of civilisation to ourselves, which are based upon a never-ending chain of misunderstandings and are trained into our nervous systems and have sunken into the unconscious.

The motoric neural pathways, also called the pyramidal tracts and the motor neurons, are the longest neural pathways in our body. Up until now it was taught that they are the pathways of our motoric intentions. With them we determine what we do with our hands and feet, but also what we do with parts of our head, the jaw and the tongue. When they have to continuously pass on a contradictory impulse, as takes place in the heel-walk, it not only affects our relationship to the world, but it also affects the second capacity of these nerves. They serve, as said, as the lesser known sensory organ, as the organ for literary sense. One can imagine the pyramidal tracts, which reach from the pyramid-shaped cells in the cerebral cortex over the spinal column into the toes, like the strings of an instrument, e.g. a guitar. Then you can easily understand what it means, when the instrument is out of tune. You then have a guitar with strings, but it's out of tune. It sounds inharmonious. It is sense-impaired. The same goes for the instrument of our body and its strings, the pyramidal tracts, our lesser known sensory organ. The learning of speech is accompanied by learning to lift – reflect – the forefoot. Ever since we were able to think, we do it with an impaired sensory organ. With general speaking habits, we lose the sensibility for this sensory disorder. In German you ask: *"Wie geht's?"* (note from the translator: *Wie geht's* means "How's it going?") No-one seems to notice that this question always addresses a process ("How does it work – e.g. the mounting of a board on the wall?"). In GODO understanding you would have to ask: "How are you going?", or "How is your IT going?"

For your entertainment – to "babble", see above – here is a small biblical excursion on which I was taken by my research: who knows whether the Babylonian history, that of urban culture with the fall of the tower, didn't actually mean the fall of the human body from the ball-gaiter to the heel-walker? In a way that people diverged as a result of it into different languages, because their literary-sense-organ suffered a sensory disorder due to an incorrect loading of the pyramidal tracts and poor posture in the entire body caused by walking in the heel-walk?

With the practice of the ball-gait, the burden to the pyramidal tracts caused by the heel-walk can be resolved. This allows the meridians to flow right down into the toes. Meridians are, after the concepts of the traditional Chinese medicine, the pathways in which the energy in our bio-electric-magnetic body flows. These were, up until now, stowed in the joints of the feet, which aren't called "fetters" for nothing. They are most strongly affected by the superfluous, counterproductive and habitual "I don't want" gesture and the "tock-tock" noise. The heel-walker lives at a minimum level of energy, mostly without noticing it. It's as if the feet are snapped off – and our feeling of connection with the energy of the earth whilst walking is like that too. At the same time, the lameness affects our tongue, which can be seen as the foot of our heart, and which would like to dance between the teeth like in a temple with thirty-two pillars. The native language learned in childhood only shows a portion of the whole original potential of language in which our tongues could gesticulate. That's why we can only communicate with each other within the limits of our language. That means that we human beings tend to lose contact with each other within the limits of language. We can bridge that by "talking with hands and feet". Woe to us if we accidentally bear swords and boots in doing so. By this stage at the very latest, you will have noticed that GODO, the ball-gait, is more than a purely physical transition.

GODO shows: We may assume that a child, who has not been misled to the heel-walk, will have hardly any fault in his upright body structure, or in his supply of energy and will also not suffer from mental disorder.

Pregnancy, Birth and the "Sensitive Phase"

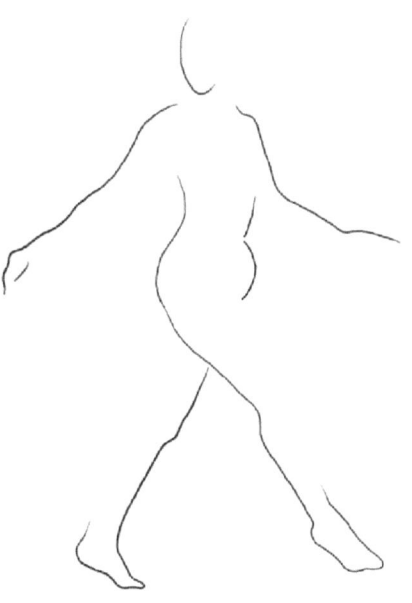

You can probably already imagine how especially meaningful and important the ball-gait is for expecting mothers, their future children and for their mutual relationships. Expecting mothers are basically the most important contacts for GODO. They should have already decided on the ball-gait before the pregnancy, at the latest before the fourth month of it. For they retain the elasticity of the pelvic floor muscles, which leads to less peritoneal tears and a less painful birth. Just imagine how the pelvic floor cramps as a reaction to the strike of the heel in every step, so that the increasingly heavier fruit of the womb doesn't fall out. This trains the pelvic floor to react with pressure from the top by holding tight in a neurotic way. When contractions then want to expel the fruit, the pelvic floor holds against it in a pointless and painful way. This makes the birth difficult for the mother and the child, in addition it can unconsciously cause a lasting conflict in the relationship between both of them, which possibly has a life-long effect (see the chapter "Regular Birth, Power – Powerlessness, Defiant Behaviour, Sexist Socialisation"). On top of that, due to the fact that the unborn child can hear at an early stage in its development, it is obvious that it can listen to the movements of the ball-gait of the "mother ship", instead of being at mercy to the sound of the bones in the heel-walk.

The **inner ear** is a threefold sensory organ. It has matured in about the fifteenth week of intrauterine development and connects itself with its central cerebral cortex between the sixteenth and eighteenth week. It is the first and apparently most important sensory organ and comprises of the three senses of **hearing, balance and gravity.** These belong very close together. If something "goes wrong" in cross-linking with the brain, it has lifetime consequences. The information coming in this "sensitive phase" becomes a kind of software, which is fundamental for all further conditioning with this sense. Whoever would like to read interesting scientific information about this, Alfred Tomatis' books are highly recommended (see the reference list). Whoever tends more towards literature, should read something by Joachim E. Berendt (as above).

So, in the womb the course is being set which determines the development of walking and talking behaviour, and thus the foundation of our ability to have balanced communication skills our whole life long. Dr A. Jean Ayres, focusing on the psychomotoric integration of children, says: "The sense of balance forms the fundamental relations that a person has to gravity and his physical environment" (*"Bausteine der kindlichen Entwicklung" ("Components of infant development")*).

The time between the sixteenth and the eighteenth week of pregnancy is called the **"sensitive phase" in the development of the sense of hearing.** The embryo now notices the walking pattern of the "mother ship" with his ears, as his three senses of hearing, balance and gravity are now fully developed. The tock-tock-tock from the chain of the mother's bones in walking on the heels is transmitted direct into the programming of the embryo's brain. The biocomputer of the unborn ball-gaiter shall bear the engram (firmly registered programme) of a heel-walker. An error creeps in with it which deeply impairs the feeling of wholeness, the integration of the individual.

For a better understanding of what can happen here, experiments made forty years ago on young kittens are being mentioned at this point. You must surely know that kittens are born with their eyes closed and open them after fourteen days. They wanted to know what would happen if the eyes of the kittens were bandaged up before they were opened, and the bandages were taken off after a further fourteen days ... The kittens were incurably blind, even though they had healthy eyes and a healthy brain. They had prevented the connecting link between the eyes and the brain at the only time in which learning to see was available in their genetic program. Thus the "sensitive phase" was discovered. All stages of development take place in such genetically predetermined times, the sensitive phase. We don't know enough about it yet. Verifiable is nevertheless, that in the minutes and hours round about the birth, there are thousands of such impressing moments. That which is omitted and impaired at this time cannot ever really be made up for.

GODO shows: move light-footed, smoothly, striding like a dancer in your muscular chain during pregnancy, then you will deliver easier.

The usual **regular birth** causes further interference of our ball-gaiting self-perception. We come namely as a premature baby into the world. It's six months after the birth that we are first fully developed. Mammals of our stage of development – like apes, horses or cows – are born mature. That's why they can stand up right after birth and be in full motion. We would have reached this stage of maturity after eighteen months. But then our head, because of the fast development of the brain, would be too big for the opening in the pelvis during birth.

It's interesting that children born under water – in contrast to people born by regular birth – start to straighten up on their own from the sixth to the eighth month of their life and soon begin to walk. Many mothers are startled by this statement because they have suffered a lot under their child's restless stage of crawling. But they don't need to be startled, as being able to stand up early is caused by a better integration of movement. The social environment is less burdened with the phase of crawling of the "mobile Me", which is often so stressful.

With the usual regular birth (premature birth), our organism has not yet evolved to the rate of gravity of which it is at mercy to in such an abrupt manner. Children react by cramping or going limp under the sudden influence of gravity. They just don't know about the conditions of gravity yet. Every movement under this completely new circumstance is strange for them. They have no control over themselves. Just bear in mind how such an insecurity in the postnatal time can influence and determine the rest of your life.

In a **water birth,** the shocks of birth, coldness, loss of balance and disorientation are mostly avoided. Us regular born children – most of us weren't born under water – took our first breath into a body which was not only extremely stressed from the birth process, but in particular from the sudden influence of gravity. In contrast, the water baby has the time and the possibility to move all its limbs in the weightlessness that's under the water with agility and in freedom. It's able to first of all find its balance, sort out its body and thus find itself again before it takes its first breath of air on the surface of the water into a then relaxed organism.

By the way, it has been discovered that in ninety-one per cent of all children, the regular birth leads to a displacement of the neck vertebrae (KISS-syndrome), which is later corrected in only thirty to fifty per cent of children by themselves. Up until now several different surgeons have concluded that this "misfortune" can and should be forestalled with a caesarean section. Obviously these doctors have never seen how water babies behave in the weightlessness of the water sluices and what they experience there. Water babies look around straight away with their eyes open and sort their neck out themselves. They are less seldom dislocated out of joint anyway, because midwives and obstetricians hardly ever have to intervene in the delivery.

Here are some additional notes on both of the main forms of birth and their effects on our vivacity.

Regular Birth, Power – Powerlessness, Defiant Behaviour, Sexist Socialisation

Regular births in the squatting position, lying down and in all kinds of birth-stools, even with the "most gentle" of births, are a very conflicting first encounter with matter, gravity and atmosphere. The encounter can, as is well known, create an extremely strong birth trauma. Such a birth, and the accidental encounter with matter connected to it, presents a shock which is seldom wholly resolved. It is like a hurt that continuously resonates later in the heel-walk. The stressful strain this reverberation generates in our connective tissue, the bearer of mental images and ideas, burdens the whole organism to an ever increasing extent over the course of a lifetime. Our connective tissue is rarely taken seriously as an organ covering the whole body, nor is it recognised for the importance it is actually entitled to. You all know it. It's exactly what you don't want on your piece of meat, that which you cut away as a tendon, or pull off as muscular fascia and throw into the bin. Even the student in the anatomical course on sectioning cleans off the muscular fascia from the muscles of the corpse, so that the specimen looks neat and tidy. The connecting tissue traverses and surrounds all of the organs like a network. It consists of simple, primary cells that work conducting electricity in a completely different way than the nerve paths. Nerves are like motorways, and connecting tissue is like green, highly communicative nature. Nerves conduct from A to B. Connecting tissue, in contrast, always knows how we are in all parts at the same time. It's the carrier of all forms of consciousness, from the skin right down into the bones. It forms the organ capsules and runs through all of the organs. It forms the tubes of the blood vessels and even the blood cells, and last but not least it supplies the cells with immune defence as well. Even blood clotting is done in the connecting tissues, as the threads of fibrin, which coil like a net in the drops of blood when it comes into contact with oxygen, originate from connecting tissue. In a way it constitutes the temple of our body and with that, the imaginary shape that we have of ourselves. I call it bearing an idea of an inner body pattern.

Birth trauma and strikes of the heels, as well as all injuries, are stored in the connecting tissue as hardening and different kinds of scarring. These forms, which instead of being possibly fluent, harden themselves, and become inner prisons, so to speak, and they define our feeling of self-worth. To remind you again: the strike of the heel, which simulates about fifty kilos of excess weight per step, adds up within the life of an eighty-year-old to the weight of the large pyramid of Giza, which we personally carry on our shoulders like the famous Atlas, or store up in our connecting tissue. This takes on some kind of gestalt in us, which I like to call the weight (note from the translator: the author wrote *"Ge(h)-Wicht"* in German, which literally translated means "go-dwarf"). By the way, the famous "devil" is really nothing less than an echo from our connecting tissue, which is created in us by the strike of the heel. Under additional stress we project this "devil" onto our fellow human beings, or we tempt providence, so to speak. In reality it is the hard core of our ego and our superego, and thus it's the main problem, that is so difficult to manage. And in being such it is the problem of social mass.

In walking on the heel, the harmony of a sense of balance is impaired by the behaviour of the feet, of the gesture of I-don't-want-to-feel, I-don't-want-to-want. In every step unconscious fear of falling is being created, making the static Me feel insecure. You remember: to prevent this feeling of insecurity the child looks for dependency and support in the psychosocial area, by developing "sails" in the form of "mental dog-ears", which we already recognised as the super ego and the ego (see the chapter "Gait and ME-development). Both figures are only fantasies of the imagination, so they don't correspond to the individual truth: they are actually only early compensations for the fear of falling, that were initially created by the resilience of the pelvic floor in regular birth and by the sudden impact of gravity. It was then confirmed from step to step with disturbed balance and "falling" onto the heels when learning to walk on the heels. This fear, an inner feeling of chaos, that smoulders deeply in every heel-walker, eventually expresses itself in our socio-political, often overly exaggerated call for institutes of order and security. (In psychology, behaviour is called "compensating" when feelings of inferiority are compensated with imagination or acts which should create the consciousness of integrity and safety. Distress becomes hidden by a virtue. Projection is a way to blame others of the own faults.)

In this context, here are a few remarks to the relation between power – powerlessness: up until now there has been a tendency to look upon powerlessness as a product of power. For me at least, it seems to be reasonable to take a look at things the other way round: Power as a compensation of powerlessness (actually every woman, or impaired femininity in men as well as in women, already knows this).

When are we most powerful in our life? As long as we are still under one year old and can neither move our body everywhere, nor talk to others using language, we possess the actuation of nurturing instinct and in doing so, we dominate grown-ups. On the other side, just bear in mind how infinitely powerful the parents appear to us, who – with the power of the heel-walk and language – can move "freely" for themselves.

If, especially during the first few months, but also beyond the crawling age, we aren't solely carried by our parents – we are namely so-called carry-babies, as Jean Liedloff verifies in *"The Continuum Concept: In Search of Happiness Lost"* – then there is extreme significance placed on the steps of the grown-ups. The steps in the heel-walk cause vibrations in the room, which signify to the child in the cradle the coming and going of the attention it gets. This can give rise to the drama of abandonment and cause psychotic disorder in all children to some degree. This psychosis is equivalent to the conflict of power – powerlessness. Whilst parents possess the apparent power of movement, there is in contrast the powerlessness of movement in early childhood. The child memorises the sounds of the steps. In this way the behavioural pattern for a whole life is designed. As soon as the set-up of its nerves is mature for walking, he will try to move in the exact same way as the grown-ups do. Then it must believe that it has the same power as the parents.

In the three-year-old child, who now believes it can walk and talk, by learning to walk on the heels, it finally translates the series of physically acted out gestures "I want – I don't want" into the mental expression of power we know as defiant disorder. (Please read this twice!)

Here is a short explanation for it: The defiant child uses "I want – I don't want" completely at random and tests the reaction of its parents. This varies, depending on the situation and according to the gender of the child and of the parent. What the father allows the daughter to do really differs from the mother's answer, and again really differs from the supposedly same requests and refusals with a male child.

I understand this sort of thing as sexist socialisation. In an emotionally disturbed heel-walking child, because of its impaired circulation system, irritated brain and the fact that it's caught in defiance, a confused understanding of the gender roles is generated. This happens during the fourth year of life. Instead of being able to integrate the undisturbed (note from the translator: the author wrote in German *"unge(h)stört"*, which literally translated means "not disrupted in walking") matured Me into the Self, we defiantly plunge, like it or not, into the oedipal sexist cultural-upbringing neurosis of our ancestors. I assume that psychologists hold their breath upon reading these words. I can only say: don't forget to breath out!

The first three years of our life and the rest of the time are obviously stored in two different spaces of consciousness, with different frames of reference. In the first space we exclusively show an interest in imitating the world. In the second space we find ourselves in the reflex of a headstrong interaction with the world. Here is the answer to your question (but perhaps you didn't have any question at all), of how could it be that before GODO no-one was aware of the fact that we are actually ball-gaiters. Significantly, in most cases we only remember back to the third year of our life. From this time on we make more and more experiences ourselves in talking and walking, which become traces of memories within us, and with which we ultimately identify ourselves as a person. At that time we started to do our very best to see ourselves as a real member of society, as social people. And in doing so, we increasingly forgot the first three years of our life.

Conscious detachment from such socialisation and the approach of a concept of the SELF as in GODO makes it difficult for a heel-walker, as you can already imagine by now, to cope with his perpetual "I want – I don't want". Methods like the Rebirthing technique of Leonard Orr, also the Holotrope Breathing of Stanislav Grof, which can bring us back into connection with the memory of our first breath, work surprisingly quick and thorough.

Water Birth

Today there have already been leading-edge and very positive experiences made with water births. They have continuously proven to be much less traumatic for the mother and child. As a result, the mother-child-relationship is less stressful right from the beginning.

Most obstetricians however see the benefits for the mother in particular (less pain), but haven't yet completely recognised the meaning of staying in the sluice for the new-born and usually take it out of the water too early.

In water, the human only has one sixth of his body-weight. The whole muscular tension, with which we have to balance the body in gravity out of the water, falls away. The pelvic floor muscles also relax. As a result, the birthing mother puts up less resistance to the delivery. Muscular activity used in the fight against gravity is eliminated by the water. The muscular pelvic floor becomes more elastic. A psychic barrier, which every mother unconsciously builds up, against letting her child, her innermost part (child, blood, water) come out unprotected into a completely strange outer environment (air, matter, gravity, light, cold) falls away.

The child develops his own spontaneous free activity under water – meaning integration before the first breath – and can unfold the limbs of his body harmonically whilst floating. It can weightlessly move its head, can look around and remember that it has come out of constriction into a greater vastness in the same warm element in which it spent nine months. In doing so, harmony in body and mind is created, which means integration before the first breath. After a few minutes in the warm vastness of water – still provided for through the umbilical cord – the child comes to the surface of the water and takes its first breath into a fully conscious and relaxed body. Such a child already learns to stand with six months of age and subsequently starts to walk earlier than a child born in the regular way. This statement can sound alarming, because the spine could possibly be burdened with straightening up too early. You have to know that this performance is possible and also brought on at exactly the right time, as the motoric integration is recovered in the sluice – proven by the conservation of the stepping reflex.

As midwives reported to me of water births, the stepping reflex is retained in children born in water up until they learn to walk. With regular born children, the stepping reflex disappears just after six weeks. I hold this disappearance as a sort of falling asleep and not as a sign of maturity. The survival of the stepping reflex points out to an undisturbed motoric integration. We regular born people really have to learn to walk again, since our stepping reflex has already gone to sleep after the sixth week of our life. In the meantime, we know that we have also forgotten our inborn ability to swim, in as much as it wasn't made possible for us as early as the first weeks of our life, or at least before the end of the first year to go to the by now proven baby-swimming. The Glottis-reflex (diving-reflex) – the automatic closure of the respiratory tract by the epiglottis – functions reflexively for four months at least until maximum the end of the first year of life, which is why no child drowns during this time.

A summary of the benefits of the water birth

Mother:

1. In water the woman giving birth only has one sixth of her body weight. This causes a full relaxation of all muscles. So no muscular tension can be built up in the supporting apparatus and the holding muscles, and in particular not in the pelvic floor muscles, impeding the delivery.

2. When a woman is giving birth, the pain of the contractions is considerably reduced just by putting her feet into warm water.

In the body-temperature full bath, about eighty per cent of the pain of the contractions are gone. Single contractions can be endured easier with their corresponding pauses. They don't lead to other muscles cramping in participation, they only take place in the uterus.

3. At the moment in time when the child is born, the mother is not as exhausted as in a regular birth. She can greet the new-born with all of her senses, completely awake and relaxed.

4. For different reasons, fifty per cent less perineal tears take place.

5. Neither infections nor drowning have been observed.

6. In most cases, mothers who have already delivered twice by caesarean sections deliver the third child with no problems in water. So-called risk-births, like the feared breech deliveries, take place "weightlessly". The half-born body of the baby swims, or floats already in the water, instead of hanging out of the birth-canal and possibly straining the cervical spine, which leads to great overall fear in the delivery room during regular deliveries.

Child:

1. Imagine how increasingly narrow it is becoming in the uterus for the growing foetus, the more the birth becomes nigh. The further passage through the "eye of the needle", the birth canal, follows after that. Imagine the feeling of becoming free into the large vastness of water after this narrowness. The newly hatched being uses the large area of the sluice to stretch out in its famil-

iar weightlessness and to move freely, whereas all contortions, e.g. of the spine, and pressures on the connecting tissues can be loosened. The narrowness is overcome. It was worth it! This feeling is taken by the child into the first breath. ("fear" and "narrowness" have the same Latin source "angus, a, um"!)

2. Reduced stress during birth, because the child has to work less against the resistance of the muscular tension of the mother's pelvic floor in the passage.

3. The warm water becomes an ideal transitional sluice. The child comes into a familiar element, where it can remember itself and in doing so, remember its development in the womb, before taking its first breath in the new, unfamiliar element of air. In this way it doesn't lose the connection to its origin. With regular birth, suddenly the world is so completely different – air, gravity, becoming touched and filling the lungs, as well as the change in the circulation – so different, that in all probability, a state of retrograde amnesia takes place, meaning forgetting caused by shock. This is obviously quite typical for all of us who were born in this way. Consider how difficult it is for you to remember the time spent in the belly of your mother. Without returning there in a therapeutic session, you can hardly attain the memory on your own. Most people even claim that such a memory isn't possible at all, even though there is enough proof for it.

4. As the child already has the eyes open in the water, it isn't immediately exposed to the whole glaringness of light, nor to the shock of cold vapour in the air. So the new-born child can look around in the water and find initial orientation – which it does very extensively if allowed enough time under water. In the wa-

ter the head of the baby isn't as heavy as on land. It can move it freely right from the start and can unfold the whole of its body. (Remember in contrast the faces of regular born babies, often contorted with pain, and understand how much they are suddenly at mercy to the all-dominating gravity. Their little head has to be held by the obstetrician.)

5. As the child doesn't get to the air immediately, no breathing reflex occurs. The glottis-reflex ensures that the epiglottis remains closed, so that no water gets into the lungs. The child is further provided for through the umbilical cord. This has the advantage that whilst swimming and being weightless, it "survives" the shock of the still relatively strenuous passage through the birth-canal, even though it was under gentle conditions, which means it can re-integrate before taking the first breath. The child regains its physical balance, its physical regulation and in doing so, it is already integrated once again; it has overcome the shock when the air fills its lungs for the first time. (In regular birth the child breathes into a twisted and stressed body, still governed by a cold-shock and at the mercy of fully unfamiliar gravity. The extreme variations of stress in regular birth can "seal" our fate as life-long disturbed birth-traumatised beings.)

6. The first caresses the baby experiences from people's hands under water are much more tender than in regular birth. (How clearly, for example, the strong grip of an obstetrician can plant an engram, meaning that it can create specific patterns of memory, is shown on a grown-up person who underwent a re-birthing session. For a short time afterwards he featured huge dark blue marks similar to marks of the obstetrician's hands on his lower legs.)

7. The earliest mother-child-relationship begins in a more tender way.

8. Warm water and patience create a much lighter atmosphere for the birth situation than all conditions of regular birth could ever produce.

9. The children develop more initiative during the course of birth.

10. Breech presentations make less problems, as the body, born before the head, can float supported by the water.

11. The children often show that they are much more content upon making their first cry.

12. The much earlier development to standing up (from the sixth month) is proof of the continuing development of balance. (With the regular birth we can never be caught as softly as the way the water catches us. We fall, at the sudden mercy of gravity, without orientation into hard, albeit very skilled hands. Apart from that, a new-born is very slippery, which is why the hands have to grip strongly in order to save it from falling. Our balance and with it our harmonic body patterns, which are stored in the connective tissue, become lost, and leave behind a distorted body. Under these poor conditions we take the first breath of air.)

Unfortunately our health system, due to its accounting procedures, discourages more children to be born under water. Water births in particular are settled as "natural births", and for this there is hardly any money, whereas caesarean sections, episiotomies, the care of wounds and bed occupancies allow a manifold fee to be made available.

The Aquatic Ape

At this point I would like to give you some information about the aquatic ape theory according to Prof. Alister Hardy, who spent his teaching career in Oxford. He correspondingly said: If, in the history of our evolution – after we had been apes – we would not already have been forced to a life in and on water for a long time, then we would still probably be just as sparsely endowed with an erect pelvis and flipper-like feet today, as our cousins, the land apes. According to Prof. Hardy's opinion, we descend from a species of African apes that was forced to live on small islands 10 to 5 million years ago. At the outset of this time, at the end of the Miocene, the large sea flooded areas of the north African continent. The ridges of the Danakil mountain range made up the islands, on which our ancestors remained imprisoned five million years long. The islands no longer permitted that our ancestors could undertake long hikes for the search of food in the plant kingdom, as they usually did. All of a sudden they were surrounded by water everywhere. That forced them to take food out of the water. Somehow they managed to adapt themselves and to survive, even though they weren't initially very good swimmers. In doing so, they benefited from the fact that the temperature of the sea was then a few degrees higher than it is today.

What powers would have been in play to finally create those mutants, which are our direct ancestors? Only on and in water did he have a niche to survive. In the Savannah, such a mutant wouldn't have been capable of surviving. The commonly known Savannah theory, after which we should have acquired the upright gait in the Savannah, just makes no sense. You can immediately understand this if you imagine that a baby ape with human feet hasn't got strong feet with claws to grip any more, to enable it to hold tight to its mother's fur. In addition to its relatively early birth, immaturity and hairlessness, such a child would have had a much too heavy head. All this would never have allowed it to survive. It was millions of years later that our ancestors could have conquered the Savannah as a habitat.

This statement will send a shiver up the back of many a "scientist", to whom the Savannah-theory is still popular (and that's most of them). It's a shame that the few who have overcome the Savannah-theory, and who campaign for a water-related development of the people of today, ultimately deny Prof. Alister Hardy, meaning they don't quote him. For such offences politicians are deprived of their doctorates.

Being in the water, his special assets brought him only advantages over the other apes. A female ape from an ape family, who (7.5 million years ago) had already lived for 2.5 million years on small islands near to the warm water, had problems to relax so deeply on land, to enable her to let go in birthing a mutant baby with a very large head. They went into the water to give birth. The little mutant baby slid into the water, and its special assets – exactly that which made them different from other apes – made them into aquatic apes: the layer of fat under the skin, which other apes don't have, gave them buoyancy and at the same time protected them from cooling off. Their upright pelvis made it possible for them to stretch themselves flat out and be carried by the water. That was the start of the weightless erecting of the body. So the erecting was easy and it also made skilful swimming in the dolphin style possible. This, as well as flipper-like feet and adverse thumbs made the aquatic apes into better swimmers and more skilful anglers, and gave them a very impressive appearance on land. They could swim better in the dolphin style and grab fish better in the gills.

As already stated, we only have one sixth of our body weight in water. This allowed the mutant person – by up to sixteen hours daily under such ideal living conditions in water – to come onto land in a very relaxed state. Such an upright "ape" emerging out of the water also received the respect of all the other apes then, who must have reacted to his uprightness as looking upon him as showing off. With apes, showing off is caused by hormones and is thus compulsive and only temporary, whereas the aquatic ape had an upright body posture available, which was genetically provided to them. Remember our reptilian morphology, the heel bone.

The thought is also very interesting, that we could only achieve the control of breathing necessary for speech acquisition with a phase of living in and on water. (You can read a lot more about this in Elaine Morgan's *Kinder des Ozeans* (*Children of the Ocean*.))

All mutants who were of a less complex and adaptable nature probably died. Therefore it seems possible to me that we ourselves are the famous missing link. Then we would be descendants of a particularly successful mutation of these first aquatic apes.

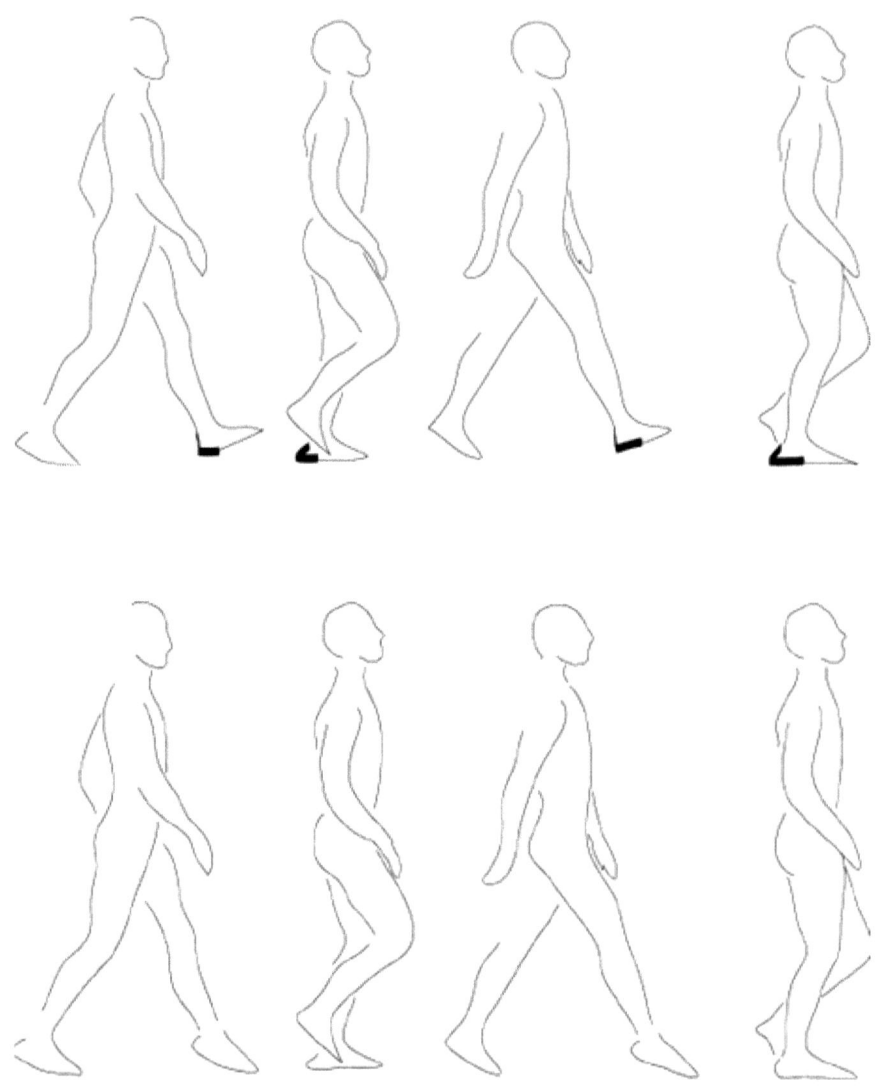

Feet, Fashion and GODO

Here is a sample of general knowledge about feet. Gerd Heinz-Mohr writes in his *Lexikon der Symbole (The Encyclopedia of Symbols)*:
"...Foot. As the lowest part on the human being, his connection to the earth, the foot has an ancient magical meaning, which is shown especially in its ritual denodation (see also Mesopotamia, Crete, Gaul). The sacrificial [...] bares his naked feet, in order to show the double relationship between heaven and earth. For the Chaldaen priest the exposing of the bare feet (pars pro toto) symbolised a form of hierogamy [which means melting with the saints]. From this point on, the frequent exposure of Moses feet on the Sinai (2nd book of Moses, v. 3,5), as well as the customary taking off of the footwear when entering a mosque [Muslims] as a demonstration of total openness and receptivity, is important for the manifestation of the divine power, just as the washing of the feet, which Jesus performs on his disciples (John 13), and ordering the apostles and the seventy disciples (Math. 10, v.10; Luke 10, v.4) to go barefoot out into the world."

Lotus Feet

The following story began in China around the year 1000 AD and ended in 1920, thanks to the Cultural Revolution, with a legal ban. At present there are still a few hundred women in China with feet mutilated in such a way, who are also still very proud of their "little lotus feet". They live on in the spirit of a past time. The last factory making shoes for them was closed just a few years ago.

For almost 1000 years, the infuriating habit existed of binding girls' feet from four to eight years of age in such a way that the toes, along with the balls of the forefoot, were ultimately located at the heels and the desired "lotus feet" were created. The mid-foot, the arches of the feet and consequently the function of movement disappeared completely with this. The bony foot becomes totally crippled. An appalling suffering in favour of an ideal of beauty.

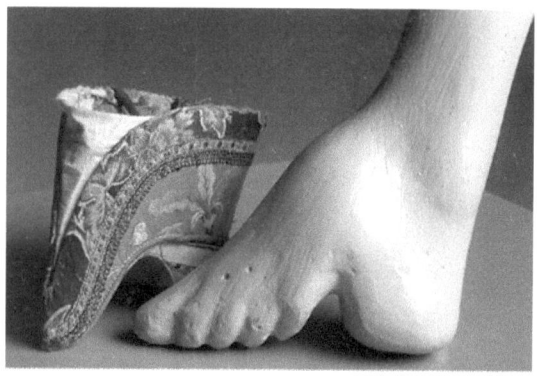

Curiously, it was these women themselves who initially took pleasure in this ideal. 1500 years earlier, around about 500 BC, there was once a Chinese empress whom the women of China remembered. They wanted to be the same as her. What the Chinese women didn't know was that this empress was born with clubfeet and in those days an ideal of beauty had been made out of her birth defect, by talking about her "tiny enchanting lotus feet". It was the women of the ruling class, who only very rarely needed to move themselves around because they had servants for everything, who inflicted torture on themselves and on their daughters. After 1500 years, while hardly any other woman was "granted" the tiny feet of the empress in an organic way, they started to mutilate themselves purely because they wanted to impress. It was favoured by the men that their women weren't able to run away, and they enjoyed the prestige when their women attracted considerable attention by coming along on their especially tiny lotus feet, supported by several female servants. A perverse nostalgic act of emancipation. The Cultural Revolution in 1919 ultimately truly freed the feet of the women.

The History of Heel Fashion

There is a very strange connection between the bad habit of the Chinese, who bound feet, and the beginning of ballet in Europe – and from this to the present heel trend. Of all people it was wild Dschingis Khan, with his close relationship to nature as king of an empire on horseback, to whom we thank the discovery of ballet. In order to understand the sensibility of such an expert horseman, you have to know that the present horse evolved from an almost shepherd dog sized, four-toed ancient horse. So the four-toed animal evolved into this wonderful one-hoofed tiptoe-walker, whose milk is most similar to human milk. It felt too restricted for the Mongolian equestrian ruler Dschingis Khan near a land like China, which had begun to mutilate women's feet. He must have deeply loathed the cult of the Chinese lotus feet. Irrespective of his feared barbarism, he was a great connoisseur. He sought the most beautiful and the tallest ones out from amongst the conquered women. Many of the applicants stood themselves up on the balls of their feet and onto the tips of their toes to make themselves appear taller to attract his attention. Legend has it that the idea of ballet came into being because of this.

A guaranteed source on the other hand, is the following history of the origin of ballet. Around 1250, after the giant realm of Dschingis Khan had long since crumbled, groups of Mongolians travelled through the whole of Europe performing theatre. At a performance of one of their ethnic equestrian dances at the Medici court, largely dancing on the balls of the feet, a princess jumped up, totally out of herself and called out rapturously: "Balleo! – I'm dancing!" This Medici travelled to Paris and created the "ballet" there for the first time. Very slowly the energy released by it spread and caused a kind of euphoria amongst people, which was expressed in round dances.

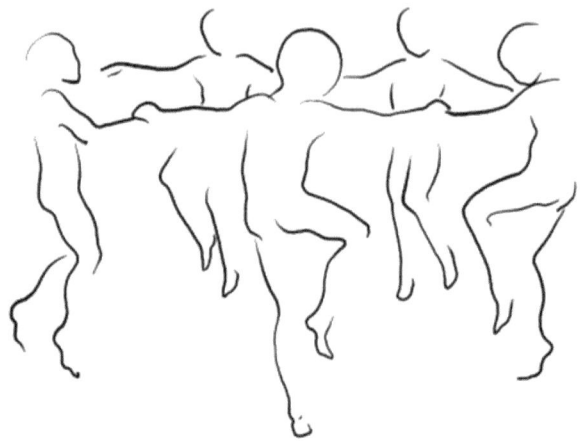

These were eventually danced in churches as well, which prompted the Vatican to ban the popular round dances by decision of the council around 1550. Eighty years later, in the middle of the Thirty Years War, ballet itself was banned by the church council. They banned it from all public stages for seventy years until 1700. During this time it was allowed exclusively "for observation" in the Jesuit monasteries in the south of France. Did the Jesuits know about the value and the effect of the ball-gait? Even Mozart was reprimanded in 1730 by the royals, because he had worked a ballet into his opera *The Marriage of Figaro*.

Some of the particularly alert and critical contemporaries amongst the nobles and the rich reacted to the ban on ballet by wearing bright red, eight to twelve centimetre high heels on their shoes, which they understood as protest against the loss of the role ballet had played. They wore these "prosthesis" when they drove through Europe in their coaches. Very few people understood its meaning. The protest was thus misunderstood as fashion. It is only since then that there are heels on shoes. (This information is based upon research along the cross-references of the Brockhaus encyclopaedia from 1956.)

Did you know that it is only since the 19th century that there have been left and right shoes? With the downfall of the Roman Empire, the knowledge disappeared of how to make shoes different. In the 17th century the shoemakers worked on leather shoes for both feet on a symmetrical moulding. And have you ever thought about what heels really do to us? Every millimetre of heel reduces two millimetres of freedom of movement. On the one hand it passively lifts us up, on the other hand it prevents us sinking down onto the flat sole of the foot. It reduces part of the spring force, weakens our will and doesn't allow us to come to rest. So heels block us both psychologically and physically. For centuries we've lost the feeling for this more and more. Today we allow ourselves more than ever to be seduced by sophisticated heel technology, aimed at reducing the impact of the heel.

In the book *Women Who Run With the Wolves*, Clarissa Pinkola Estés wrote:

"In the south-west of the united states the wise old women are also called, amongst other things, LA QUE SABE, the knower. I heard about the knowers for the first time when I lived in the Sangre de Christo mountains of Santa Fe, where an old Mexican woman told me that LA QUE SABE had made the sexual organ of women at the beginning of creation from a crease in her divine foot-sole.
That's the reason, the old woman meant, why women are normally clever: after all they are essentially made from the highly sensitive skin of the sole, which feels everything, everything at the same time! The idea that the skin of the sole could serve as a sensitive perceptive organ was confirmed to me by a squaw from the tribe of Kiché. She told me that she had to wear a pair of shoes for the first time at the age of twenty, but she could never get used to them – con los ojos vendados –, nor to walking through the world with blindfolds on the feet."

How do I learn GODO quickest?

*"The only true power,
over which we ultimately dispose of,
is the power to change ourselves for the better."*

Gabrielle Roth:
Maps to Ecstasy

*"It is a matter of slowly switching the awareness.
Lifting the free leg and balancing so long that a new walk comes out of it!"*

Matthias Horx:
How we will Live: A Synthesis of Life in the Future

As a Ball-Gaiter you will become the Person you are

Before every new "learning to walk", everyone should be clear about the ideal functional position of his feet. For this purpose, stand with your feet shoulder-width apart. A lot of people stand with the tips of the feet pointed outwards. This breaks the axis of your uprightness and at the same time causes splayfeet, flatfeet and abducted feet. Feet placed parallel to each other also rarely comply with the shape of the human foot.

Look closely at how feet are constructed. How does the line of the primary joints of your toes run in regard to the walking direction? We should actually walk and stand with feet placed lightly inwards, just as babies take their first tiny steps. Do you remember? Standing always comes before walking, so it's important to exercise the right position here.

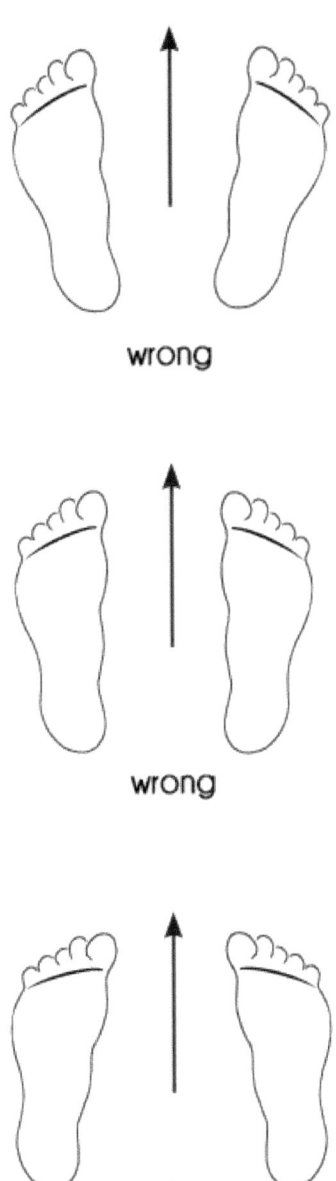

The primary joints of the toes only function
as unbroken hinges in this position

If you push your knees through, then you're blocking all dependent joints: ankles, hips, pelvis and the lower back. So please always stand with lightly opened knee-joints.

If you push the opened knee-joints lightly to the outside whilst standing in the right position with your feet, you shift your weight onto the outer edge of the feet, and your knee-joints come into the best position, because it's the most natural one. Now the washout of the joint functions normally with the fluid in the joint, which prevents the cartilage from wearing out. In this position, move your pelvis carefully to the front and to the back. Place a hand onto your lower back whilst doing so and feel how flexible you now are.

GODO guides you not only to the right use of your feet, but to a new, swinging straightening up and a correct use of your whole body on all the levels of your joints as well.

The New Footwear

Of course we need appropriate footwear: it should have a heelless, soft sole and leave the forefoot lots of room. The big toe has to be able to show straight ahead! **If you have a barefoot feeling in your footwear, then it's right!** All real "barefoot shoes" are non-orthopaedic footwear. They hinder the development of orthopaedic problems.

In order to be able to learn and practice GODO easily, consider heelless, thin, highly flexible soles. Thereby the last phase of every step, putting the heel down until standing, can also be consciously felt. Any millimetre high heel (also hidden) is hindering for "coming to rest" into the "zero position".

My friend Martin Adam (Tel.: +49 7565/914296; www.erdspiritualitaet.de) makes custom-made footwear of all kinds out of naturally tanned leather, including the so-called peasant shoes. These feet-companions are especially suitable for children, as children's feet are particularly sensitive, and walking barefoot would actually be most suitable for their development. Unfortunately that isn't always possible. The peasant shoes from Martin Adam, with their very thin soles, offer a compromise. They convey the feeling of direct contact with the ground and support the feet and leg muscles, whilst nevertheless protecting the small feet.

Nowadays there are all sorts of colourful interim solutions in every shop selling natural products, as well as with more select specialist retailers.

Now to the Practice ...

If suitable footwear is not available, please practise each single step barefoot.

If you have the feeling that you are a rather weak-minded person, begin extensively with the phase "I want". At the same time, if you hold yourself to be especially strong-willed, you can begin with concentrating on lifting the heel, and at the same time saying or thinking "I want". In doing so, a very welcome effect will occur: after just a few steps you will become a ball-gaiter, because with particular concentration on the positive intentions, you automatically forget your heel-walking conditioning of lifting the tip of the foot, the gesture of "I don't want". That's a trick that the strong-willed heel-walker in particular should use to prove to themselves how easy it is to let go of these unnecessary, negative gestures.

Bear in mind that it's about the straightening of your body posture and enjoy being in the world with a "grateful" vagrant heart. Imagine that your legs would be the pendulums of your heart. Throw your heart into the wind and think of Charles Aznavour: LET YOURSELF GO!

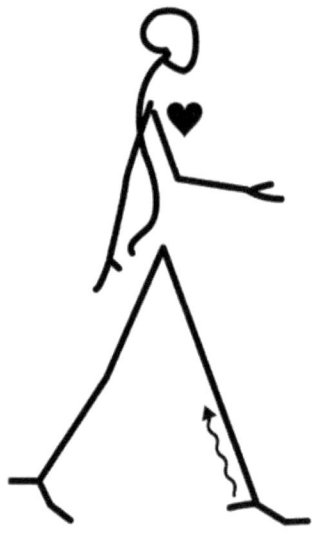

The effect of "I feel" is gotten spontaneously by everyone. We appear to experience being in a loving relationship with the earth.(Note from the translator: the author wrote *ge(h)fuehlt* which means felt in going.) Every step is heartfelt focus, the echo of which moves through our cardiovascular system.

For people laden with stress, it's recommended to start with concentrating on lowering the heel, with the "I come to rest". Taking a small, slow step backwards, you can feel the release and letting go in the joints of your feet very well. The best thing to do is to control yourself in the mirror.

Observe yourself going down stairs. You do that quite automatically in perfect GODO. In fact you only need to proceed exactly as your foot arrives from the last step on the stairs.

What's more: observe with which part of your foot you touch the pedals in riding a bicycle. Congratulations if it's the forefoot (balls of the foot), as then you already have a favourable anticipation of the ball-gait. Apart from that, it's a sign of mental alertness.

For the case that you may not make up your mind immediately to change over to the ball-gait in public, indulge once or twice a day in five minutes of some barefoot-exercises:

1. Loosen your feet in the ankles (note from the translator: "*Fesseln*" in German can be translated as "chains"). In loosening, stand up, taking turns on one leg after the other and dangling the foot of the loose leg. Change sides a few times, so that you can loosen up easier. Should you lose balance, look for support.

2. "March" on the spot with loose joints of the feet before going to sleep and after getting up. In this way you can feel into the naturalness of the movement of the ball-gait. The two halves of your brain are adjusting in doing so (hemispheric synchronisation) and this allows you to have a deeper sleep, or to be more awake. Don't forget turning the shoulders in opposite directions in this exercise. All of your spinal column joints start to dance in the process. A tip for the teachers amongst you: doing this exercise before teaching begins brings tranquillity and concentration to the class!

3. You can also make this exercise a little more imaginative. Take small single steps in all different directions: sidewards, backwards, diagonally, forward, to the right and left; stepping one foot over the other one and turning on the spot. All in constant change.

4. Jump on the spot: high, high, high and optionally, a bit forwards, sidewards and back. Stay elastic in the knees.

5. A psycho-dynamic exercise can be very helpful too. Imagine for yourself, whilst still lying in bed, how a striding walk gives you the sensual feeling of straightening up in the whole body.

The diversity of information that you have encountered here has only one major reference point, GODO, the ball-gait. I would like to provide your consciousness with as many pieces of information as possible, so that no feeling of resignation can set into your flesh and bones.

Any possible resistance to GODO may be there for a number of reasons. I would like to list a few of them:

1. For most of us, habits are difficult to give up. In the matter of the heel-walk, we are unfortunately all creatures of habit.

2. When it comes to letting go, we react with doubt and hold on tightly to the old instead.

3. The psychosocial meaning of the heel-walk is one of the most difficult adjustments in everyone's childhood, and only the thought of trying to give it up can cause major confusion.

4. Special preferences in footwear fashion which the individual has formed, in order to – so he believes – signal his special personality, are ironically often fanatically defended, particularly then when they are associated with the greatest sacrifices (painful feet, injuries, narrowness, foot deformation, back pain).

5. The fear of attracting attention: "What will the others think of me?" According to the principle of: "What does that look like?!", or: "I'm not gay!" (to my astonishment I hear this over and over again from men and women).

That's why upon reading this book it can come over and over again to insinuations like: "Why should I walk GODO now of all things, when no-one else does?", or: "Up until now I walked so well!", or: "I have to first of all wear my shoes out in the old way!", etc.

I hope that your insight will be stronger and that you can choose to walk GODO on a day of your choice. Then take a period of at least three months, in which you try to take every step in GODO awareness. You will forget it over and over again in the beginning and you will often fall back into the old routine. Don't blame yourself if that happens. You have all the time you give yourself for it.
Regard it as a game you play with yourself.
Every step is yours!
Go inside yourself!
Come out of yourself!
Experiment instead of imitating!
Admit to your own highest personal nature, the nature of the cells in your body! You are a Natio (the Latin word *"natio"* means "birth" in German). You are the Nation of your body- cells.

A small problem should additionally be mentioned here. With the ball-gait you automatically straighten yourself up better, the hips swing much more freely and the counter-turning movements of the shoulder girdle and the pelvis are also more pronounced. That's where shame can come upon us. Subjectively, we imagine ourselves as being too noticeable. Objectively though, no-one notices it in a negative way. Therefore enjoy it, just amuse yourself and stay true to your decision! In this way you can experience a daily non-stop meditation, in which you don't have to withdraw from daily happenings into silence, as is required in many other forms of meditation.

Taking a period of one year is ideal, because then you really have enough opportunity to experience the first positive effects, and develop such a great sensitivity, that afterwards you will be downright sorry for every step you took on the heels. And another small warning: when you are once sensitised for GODO, you will feel great compassion when you suddenly notice on all side-walks and pavements just how much people hurt themselves with the heel-walk.

Saint Francis, a barefoot walker, once said: *"It doesn't benefit you to go praying if your walking isn't already a prayer."* You see: the wise said what everyone knows, and the wisdom is so simple that no-one wants to believe it.

The Practical Success of GODO

GODO teaches us the upright gait, the ball-gait. In the process, the body sensations we have forgotten about return, causing a feeling of well-being. At this point I would like to emphasise that I make no healing promises, even if it may seem so in the following text. May everyone gather experience in their own way.

GODO makes the reactive patterns of movement caused by the heel-walk disappear. We are freed from the defective programming of our connective tissue. The fields of the connecting tissues – just like echoes – contain many memories of shocks caused by walking the wrong way (the heel-walk has to be endured as a wrong example as early as in the womb). This is avoided with GODO. Mothers who stride in the ball-gait don't create this problem in the first place. Pregnant women practising GODO create an elastic environment for the unborn child, their bodies resonate more harmonically, so that the development of the connections of the senses of balance, gravity and hearing in the unborn foetus can take place more harmoniously.

With double muscle pumps, GODO can reduce and even prevent many complaints of the veins.

With an improvement in the blood circulation and an activation and harmonisation of mobility, GODO can remove superfluous pounds of weight easier.

GODO alleviates arthritis.

GODO helps with damaged discs caused by bad posture, solves problems in the muscular-skeletal system; the weak back becomes strong and elastic.

GODO regulates hollow feet, flat feet, splay feet and abducted feet by the active use of the feet in striding and prevents the development of such in childhood.

Those who walk GODO don't twist their ankle quite so easily. I have never twisted my ankle since walking GODO.

GODO allows us to use our energy more ergonomically even whilst doing heavy manual work. Injuries are more seldom in the muscular and skeletal system.

GODO can prevent the tearing of Achilles tendons. The athlete who doesn't know about GODO yet, walks during his pause from training for a couple of weeks in the normal heel-walk, in which he uses his Achilles tendons only in rolling the foot and not in putting down the foot. When the athlete comes back out of the break again, partially trained in this way, it can happen that his Achilles tendon tears within the first half an hour. Statistics show that eighty per cent of all Achilles tendon tears happen under these circumstances.

GODO can prevent perspiring feet – which many people affected with it have already confirmed. The famous "athlete's foot" could soon belong to the past.

GODO can slowly free us from the unconscious fear of falling by harmonising our balance.

GODO harmonises movement, breathing, circulation and last but not least sexuality.

GODO helps to curb asthmatic attacks and often makes asthma completely disappear.

GODO synchronises both halves of our brain (hemisphere-synchronisation). This is kinesiologically verifiable.

GODO spontaneously promotes our well-being and makes us more dynamic.

GODO prevents certain types of ageing because it makes us more elastic, calmer, more able to concentrate and more active.

GODO accomplishes – as in dancing, only more constant – the harmonisation of the male and female energies in the organ of our emotional body, the circulatory system.

GODO is the ideal way of meeting asphalt with a springy, elastic step. Bear in mind that this hasn't occurred to you yet. Instead you let yourself be conned into buying heel technology (air and jelly padding) in training shoes.

With GODO, patients found out that those who inclined to allergies, had marked improvement.

Even with acute depression, but also with psychotic phases, the shear memory of GODO and a few steps in the ball-gait helped some of the affected.

GODO must always remain a free individual choice. Don't try to want to educate anyone and especially not your children to GODO. Your children only need you to go striding ahead in the GODO manner. Walk GODO at least for all the very small children who are in prams or in their parent's arms, or for the children from the first to the third year in their life, who are living at the level of your legs and who copy the way grown-ups walk.

If you decide to practice GODO out of pure love, you too will profit from it. Your real quest and chance lies here. Walk – yes, step on your forefoot showing a GODO example!

GODO Fitness

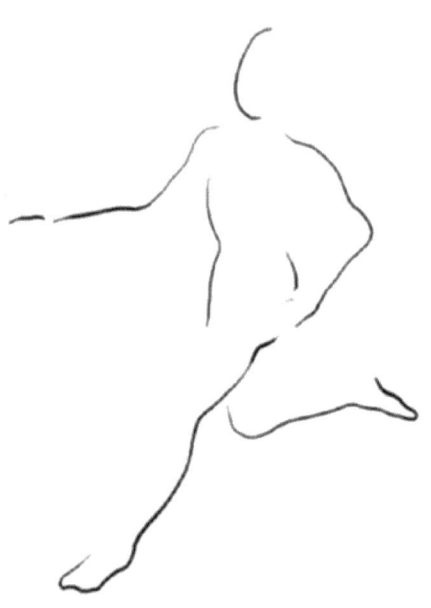

GODO is extremely important for all people who like going to fitness centres. It's important for the instructors in sport and fitness centres, as well as for all those who train in these centres, or at home on machines, as with GODO on its own, we reach a sensitivity that we can call "emotional awareness". This emotional awareness in walking is a guarantee for mental efficiency, which for the effects of physical training can be compared to the salt in the soup.

As long as the heel-walker isn't at least aware of GODO, he hasn't yet communicated to his body that he is actually designed for the ball-gait. He masters his body with the wrong program. He insults the intelligence of his body. The information about GODO on its own allows the body's intelligence to recover.

In earlier chapters I have shown: the information that GODO can relax the body in such a way that allergies, generally known as the manifestation of being marginally stressed out, disappeared, even without the consequent transition from the heel-walk to the ball-gait. Just as so-called ADHS children suddenly come to rest when they aren't devaluated any more, but are accepted in their own distinct ways, your body reacts in this way too when you confirm it in its genetic reality as a ball-gaiter.

Here is a short, critical observation on Nordic Walking, which is practised everywhere today: indeed, how can we import the summer training of northern cross-country ski runners (in which the forefeet are bond, which forces them into an expressive sliding step with an emphasis on the forefoot) as a new "exercise in marching" on the heel?! And such a thing is supported by sickness insurance companies – oh pardon me, naturally by the "health insurance companies"! Today you sometimes hear that it was due to incorrect translation. That almost sounds like an apology. I could accept it, if in taking a look at the Nordic-walkers, I could make out that they are reforming to ball-gaiters. On the other hand, I continuously witness "certified" Nordic walking trainers who react in a downright indignant manner when I try to inform them of this.

A Report based on Experience out of my Practice

Towards the end of this book, I would like to describe an incident which, as a whole, cannot be captured very easily. Read it just like a fairytale, perhaps a few times over, as then the different levels in it will slowly become clear to you.

The Miraculous Healing of an Eight-year-old Boy

It's about Sina, an eight-year-old Persian boy. After his birth he was troubled with neurodermitatis for two years. After that the neurodermitatis disappeared, but, as is often the case, it was replaced with not less unpleasant asthma. Medical science is aware of the typical course of this illness. Within the course of the last six years, Sina had to be taken to the nearest hospital with flashing blue lights because of particularly serious asthma attacks, in which he threatened to suffocate.

I got to know his father during the time I worked in a practice for natural medicine within healthcare tourism in a hotel in the Greek part of Cypress. At the reception a very quiet man of oriental appearance was on night duty. It was Sina's father. When we met, it was more glances than words that we exchanged. He spoke little and when he did, then very slowly and with intent, however in surprisingly good English. I needed some time to perceive how much he had to tell. It soon turned out that he and his family were only spending time in Cypress seeking asylum.

He came from a distinguished Muslim family – and even though he had been one of the best known national football players and one of the best students of his Persian homeland, before surviving a dreadful war as a general of the Mujahidin, he had to leave his land in haste in order to only just escape the revenge of the Mullah regime and its fundamentalist henchmen. He had studied English already before Sina's birth with the help of the Bible during a study visit to Cypress, and he was converted to Christianity five years ago with his wife and their two sons, without broadcasting about it. After some of the Moslem friends of his family saw the Bible lying around his house in Tehran, they abruptly stopped visiting them. Shortly after that he was given notice from the bank in which he had worked for years as a popular manager. He subsequently wasn't able to find work anywhere. At length he wanted to part from luxury items like cars and televisions purely to survive. He put advertisements in the newspaper to sell them and found buyers easily. Nevertheless they all brought everything back the next day and asked for their money back, because they didn't want to keep anything from a believer of another faith.

The family didn't have any other choice but to flee immediately, and so they landed in Cypress with a few former Christian fellow students of the father of the family.

The family had to be content with a one-room flat, as is often the case when one is a refugee. The father worked for the past three years on building sites or in a marmalade factory and in the nighttime there, where I met him. The mother, a high school teacher, became a seamstress in a clothing factory. Sina and his ten-year old brother, despite everything or perhaps even because of this very challenging situation, progressed during these three years to become the best scholars in their classes in the Greek school. They spoke and wrote three languages fluently.

I found all this out before the father told me about his younger son's asthma and asked me to treat him once to balance him with the bio-resonance technique, a further development of electro-acupuncture. I had already seen Sina twice for a short time when he accompanied his father to the hotel. He was a delicate, very lively and extremely bright boy with the handsomeness of an oriental prince.

Suddenly the high-tech character of the bio-resonance machines, and their impenetrability at the same time, seemed to me to be absolutely unacceptable for such a child. I didn't want to try to encounter this bubbly intelligence like a magician with a black-box, without really being able to find out what works. So I suggested to the father that I would work with the boy with GODO during an afternoon at his home. I explained to him that I needed the cooperation of both parents for this. In doing so, I would tell the whole family a long story. He would have to promise me his own concentrated attention and that of his wife, so that the children, swept along with them, would also be attentive. The constraint of having only one room should comply with my wishes.

We arranged an appointment for the next Saturday. His wife prepared a wonderful traditional Persian meal with real basmati rice for lunch. In the morning we first of all took part in the service for refugees, a set-up that on the one hand serves to create a more intimate relationship with the Cypriots, and at the same time helps them to become worthy of a reference for resettlement and admission into a country of destination.

After church we walked along the sea promenade. Here I used the chance to speak to Sina for the first time. I demonstrated my way of walking on the forefoot to him, which immediately brought him to compete with me in a striding heel-walk. He simply shot away from me in huge strides with a bent upper torso, rolling his feet off over the heels. That looked very bustling and somewhat like Donald Duck. I congratulated him on his performance and we talked about other things which I don't remember now.

Arriving at home, we sat down around the table, and while the meal was being served, the father inaugurated me into the Persian drinking ritual. He poured me a large glass of highly alcoholic grape spirit on ice, with a glass of Coca Cola to go with it, also on ice. I wanted to refuse, because I hadn't drunk any alcohol for years. But then I learnt what a real Sari is. He explained to me that I didn't need to worry, as he himself was nominated as one of the youngest Saris of the whole of Persia when he was only sixteen years old. The Saris are drinking masters. *"If a society of men want to drink, then to begin with you look for a Sari. He guarantees that all will get home safely, no matter how tough the going gets. The Sari sits at the end of the table and pours for everyone. He determines also that someone who believes he has had enough to drink still keeps on drinking, so that the whole round can continue in further upward spiralling spirit. At the end all are brought home safely by the Sari."*

I let myself in with the master and ate the rice, of which every single grain seemed to dance on my tongue, whilst I slowly began to tell the story about GODO, the striding walk on the forefoot. My hosts really pricked up their ears and on their behalf they revealed that they had actively practised yoga together five years long before their marriage, and were now admittedly sad to have neglected it during these difficult times.

The conversation didn't remain one-sided, the information flew back and forth, and the children were in full swing. Sina wanted to leave the table a few times to demonstrate his yoga skills. He had to be patient until the meal was over, but then we could all be kept still no longer. Everyone demonstrated their exercises. The father and the children mastered all sorts of very convincing techniques of falling down and getting up. Everyone began to explain his skills and listened attentively to the explanations of the others. So I had no problems to find enough hearing and full understanding for GODO. All of them practised it with me. For hours on end we had a fling with the craziest steps and other exercises, whilst the Sari always vigorously topped me up. When the children had been in bed for a long time, he brought me back to the hotel to sleep, and I accompanied him on the night shift at the reception.

Since this afternoon Sina has never had another asthma attack; although he didn't even become an active ball-gaiter. Apparently the information on its own healed him from his original way of walking. A week after our meeting he gave me a small picture that he had made himself. His mother told me that he tinkered with different variations of it for days and all were thrown away, until he was at last pleased with this picture. I have shared it here in the original size.

It shows Sina before and Sina afterwards. For this you have to know that the Persians write from the right to the left of the page and also consequently depict other logical procedures in an unusual way, which appears for us the other way round! Sina describes his release from imprisonment in a three-fold net-like captivation, which is mirrored in his asthma. It seems to me to be a self-imagined portrayal of his asthmatic condition on the level of the connective tissue. In this context you can recognise the connecting tissue as a bearer of patterns of ideas in the body. Apparently solely the information that we are not actually born as heel-walkers liberated him from these patterns of ideas in his body. The exuberant exercises during that afternoon fully integrated him.

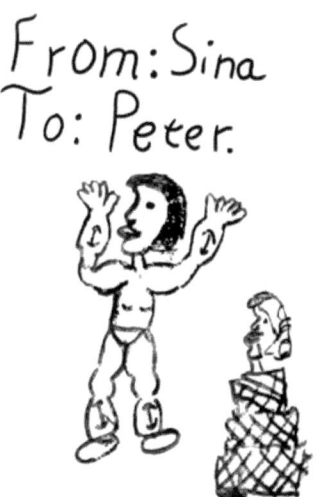

The family finally moved to Canada and they live there happily and they are healthy.

Experiences with GODO

Out of my GODO Diary
– Ellen Schernikau –

4th March 1996: I frequently notice that walking quickly in the ball-gait is difficult for me. The spiral counter-rotating movements of the body helps me tremendously to nimbly get on and furthermore conveys a feeling of pleasurable awareness – and nevertheless, I would rather walk GODO slowly. In stepping quick I always still have the impeding feeling of the backward motion, even though I've practised for almost a year. Of course I move forwards, but the rolling off from the front to the back seems to be a contradiction. Is the heel-walk more logical?

Logic back and forth: I'm all right, since my operation on a slipped disc I always had pain, since GODO I have no pain any more, and that's what's most important! And as I understand the concerns and the meaning of GODO, I now ask myself the question: why do I actually want to walk quickly? Apart from the few unavoidable occasions that make me rush, I could by all means walk slowly for most of the time – that is: perceiving, feeling, enjoying, relaxing, being here! That's why I don't want to annoy myself any longer with a supposable incapability, but do what I can, and do it with pleasure.

9th May 1996: Time's getting short, I have to catch the train. My step becomes quicker, and suddenly I perceive a constant tock-tock which goes right up into my skull – I involuntarily fall back into the heel-walk whilst walking quicker. I'm terribly annoyed about it. Just before reaching my destination, the station, I see that there is enough time. I stop and stand, become really quiet, feel the ground through the soles of my feet and ask it for forgiveness. I kiss it with my feet, do a few exercises on the balls of my feet, breathe calmly and tell myself: I will look after you just as I look after myself. Erect, I walk GODO, and I feel good again.

4th August 1998: I reflect on a fault in the sense of the wording. "Would you do me a favour?" – How often is this request spoken! A request that basically is a "trap". For: who likes to refuse a request? "It depends", is sometimes the reply, but one is nevertheless willing to do something for the other person, one wants to be nice, to be useful. "To please" means, so to speak: "go and fall (into uncertainty?)" (note from the translator: to please is in German "gefallen". The author writes "Geh-fallen", which literally translated means "go and fall"), or: "walk into my trap." The request is actually also a demand: "be bribed!" It's a contract, even before the person asked knows of its content: "If you want to please me, then do me a favour!"

To "I don't want": this statement is a contradiction in itself. "I want" means: look in front, think ahead, I have something to do, I intend to do something. With the "I don't want", I negate something positive. For example: "I don't want to argue" would be better expressed with "I am peaceful" or "I want to talk to you in peace". When the relationship between mother and child is developed on this basis, the child will be more specific. Instead of saying "I don't want cauliflower", he will now say "I don't like cauliflower."

20th March 2000: I walk GODO for five years now. Admittedly with a few fall-backs. What a shame that I didn't know what I know now before the birth of my son.

The Experience of Oneness in Walking
– Thomas Merkentrop –

Indian stories about such wonderful experiences have always fascinated me. Apart from that, there was the deactivating of the inner dialogue, which is attainable by nothing simpler than walking and "the gaze of the owl" (looking far ahead in a wide radius)! Great! So I spent an intensive time with walking and – frustration.

Even though there were wonderful moments with the heel-walk in my attempts at oneness, no absolute feeling of it came about, as I always paid too much attention to the walking, and what's more, I had to still think very, very much as well. Thereby I could really "softly" roll off over the heel (oh dear, the finger-in-the-ear-test took away the last illusion of "softly" from me), but what an effort it was. They bear no relation to each other. Something had to become different, rather, the walking had to become different.

My masterpiece was definitely the purchase of Indian moccasins, along with the question "why do my knees suddenly hurt so much?", whereby I was naturally "hacking" on my feet. Indeed exactly this led me to the ball-gait. For if you are in any way sensitive, it doesn't even seem possible to walk on the heels with moccasins on without getting aches and pains after ten minutes at the latest.

So my feet showed me "my walk!" Since then the most wonderful stories have been told: my knees are fit again and my whole body revels in best health. In the ball-gait my nose becomes free, allergies stop abruptly and I am immediately centred. But it must be said to this, that I always walk on the balls of the feet. If these little miracles would also have come about "now and again – just from time to time", I don't know. For me, super experiences showed up after about two weeks, exactly at the time when the ball-gait had become "normal". What looked like stalking in the beginning, became floating and dancing after only a few days. Just fantastic! Oh yes, and the experiences of oneness: (almost) always when I walk through the nature reserves in the twilight (it's most easiest then, that's the time in-between the worlds, try it sometime), I melt with the surroundings and a feeling of peace touches my heart. It's as if the voices of nature revel in me.

Readers' Letters

"There is a simple pattern.
Ask someone about his ideal
and ask him about the reality.
If he starts to sing about his ideal, you're off.
If he starts to moan about his reality, forget it."

Ronald M. Schernikau

Dear Doctor Greb,

Since we met in the summer of 1998 a lot has happened. I am the small sixty-year-old photographer from Kiel, and we met at a sitar-concert in Johannes Loeffler's place at the Zentrum Oase. At the time you rendered your thoughts on GODO and presented a good example with your own appearance. It took about six weeks until I mastered GODO completely harmoniously, and without falling back into the old sixty-year-old practice of walking I had. I didn't tell you then that I am seventy per cent invalidated. My pelvis was shattered several times in a car accident and a central hip luxation has led to a difference of four and a half centimetres in the width of the pelvis in my side. As a dancing and gymnastic teacher and physiotherapist, I became unable to work because of it. Since this accident twenty-five years ago I was never free of pain. Due to my physical awkwardness I got a heel bone fracture in five pieces five years ago, which is relatively well healed up. Over the years I had gotten painful, somewhat bent hip joints and walked slightly bent over. I couldn't run any more. The doctors actually only allowed me to walk one kilometre each day.

With walking GODO I immediately felt much more elated and had a far better mood, as I could somehow straighten myself up more. I moved forward quicker, my legs became stronger and I was more nimble on the ground, which I had always found extremely difficult when I was taking photographs of children and animals. With the accident my legs felt different in length, which I had balanced out up until now with a straight and a slightly bent knee. Now I walk more evenly and stretch both legs the same. With the forefoot-step my steps seem to be bigger, I balance the difference in the length of my legs with steps of different lengths. I run again, dance Tango and take part in a folk dancing group. Not so long ago I walked fourteen kilometres over the mountains in Bund shoes from Martin Adam. In the last two years I feel years younger. My professional work as a photographer has increased in creativity and success.

Thank you most sincerely!
Ute Boeters, Kiel, 2000

I would like to add a few experiences from the last years between 2000 and 2014:

In the summer I walk barefoot, first of all only because I can walk quicker and safer up and down the four floors in my house with naked feet, and because I can kneel down easier when taking photos on the ground. My big toe, slanted outwards by the Hallux-valgus, the bunion I have, noticeably straightened itself out. Walking barefoot is for me the only logical result of GODO. The feet touch down on the ground very flat in a groping-like manner with the balls of the little toes first. In doing so my toes fan out and lift themselves somewhat from the ground. Shortly after, the balls of the big toes touchdown and finally the heel comes. It's only when transferring my weight, that the tops of all the toes grip the ground.

I know other barefoot walkers who walk on the heels, with scorfed skin on the soles of their feet, cracked on the edges of the heel and bloodily chapped. I now wanted to know if I would also get horny skin walking with GODO. I didn't get any. My feet are completely smooth and they always feel warm. Thick muscles grew underneath of my feet. My toes stretched out. The soles of the feet sometimes feel hot and tingly, as if fur skin would be growing under them. I walk with pleasure over cool, smooth tiles.

My shoes have all been given away. The foot caps pressed my toes painfully together and the thick muscles on the soles of my feet only waged war against the foot-bed in them. The fact that thick, hard skin only results from abuse (the heel-walk), can be demonstrated on my feet. Only my big toe developed an edge of hard skin on the crooked spot. If it would be straight, I wouldn't abuse it. The skin on the whole of the soles of my feet is so nice and smooth that it shines and always looks clean. I don't even put cream on them. Isn't that another further scientific proof that we are born as ball-gaiters?

For more than twelve years now I walk barefoot the whole year round, also in snow, even if it's only to the bins, the woodshed, the letterbox round the corner or to the car. I drive barefoot and usually ride bicycle barefoot. When I have to sweep snow round my house, or if there are pieces of glass lying on the path when there has been a public festival, then I put on barefoot Leguanos. I can only safely walk the four floors in my house barefoot. Due to the forefoot-gait I have gotten calves which remind me again of my body as it was during my time as a dance and sports teacher. In comparison to then, I notice that my balancing capacity has clearly developed so much muscular strength and body economics with GODO, that I can now stand a lot better on the balls of my feet with seventy-five years of age and I'm as centred and balanced as I am dancing the tango.

Two and a half years ago my hip joint, which was damaged in the accident, became more awkward. At least it had held out for thirty-nine years. Pain, caused by all sorts of relieving postures I used to help me escape the feeling of dragging around trousers made of iron, was now not only just in the groin any more, but strangely enough in the back, on the other knee or in the shoulder. My leg became thinner and caused instability on walking the stairs. A walking aid took away some of the pain, but the muscles diminished even quicker. On the extreme tips of the toes, I could, to my surprise, walk quite pain-free. The stairs were also taken easier with this balanced tension in the muscles near the joint. I used my Bellicon several times a day now for balancing exercises to train these muscles. As nothing else worked, an endoprosthese was implanted.

After three weeks doing my barefoot exercises in GODO terms on the Trimilin, I was completely fit for work again. My training in advance with the ball-gait and the exercises afterwards in warm water helped me very much.

Ute Boeters
info@fotoatelier-boeters.de

Dear Dr Greb,

I have just finished reading your book and would like to order another three of them from you – to lend and to display. Up until now I have always encouraged my patients to walk, because for me it is the most worthwhile form of movement – now it is GODO. It's remarkable that everyone notices the lightness. I like it very much. Thank you very much.

Warmly,
Sylvia Pietrzok, Neukirchen

Dear Peter,

You asked me if I would like to say something about GODO, and on the spur of the moment I enthusiastically said yes!
So: GODO ... and what it really means for me? Getting to the heart of it – is a difficult undertaking!

What has changed? I think this is a good starting point: it's been six years since a cheerful, loving person with an outrageously long beard came into my life. And along with him came GODO. Basically quite easy to learn, but for me with all the years of control I've acquired and this tension, it was a real challenge. All of a sudden it was required of me to let go. First of all just in the feet, yet before I knew it, my whole body tried to go along with it. The pelvis, the lower abdomen, the shoulder region ... It wasn't only the beginning of a different sense of body awareness, no, of my emotional and intellectual patterns too, which revealed themselves in this bent position, with lightly drawn up shoulders and purely thoracic breathing, and suddenly it got into a flow. A lot in me struggled tooth and nail against this straightening up, which demanded a confrontation with many repressed, partly painful issues, or with the things I had been holding under control!

In the end it took a few years until I had really implemented GODO into my daily life. Now during my pregnancy I have become aware of the value of GODO again: the pain, especially in the lower back, which bothers many pregnant women, disappears in a wondrous way after a few steps GODO. Even in the last month of pregnancy my gait appears to be relatively light-footed and it still gives me pleasure to be active. It's especially nice to experience the feeling of letting go in the belly when I stride in this way: my baby is swayed gently to and fro, and the blow in the lower abdomen with every step in the heel-walk is just gone!

GODO ... and what it really means for me: GODO means conscious awareness for me. To become conscious inside of myself and to become conscious with the outside of me! It is so wonderful to walk GODO barefoot on the beach in the summer and to touch mother earth very gently and lovingly with the feet!

Thank you! Love,
Sinje, naturopath, Hamburg
sinje.hansen@web.de

Dear Peter,

I would sincerely like to thank you today, that I was able to participate in one of your GODO workshops. Since then I have gotten a wonderful new feeling for my body and have come to know and love it. With the right use of my feet I feel light and floating. Fear of pain in the skeletal-system now belongs to the past. With the knowledge I acquired from you, I have become my own best friend.

With the wish that you can still teach many people to have a positive body awareness, just as you have helped me, I remain with kind regards.

Gisela, Karlsruhe

Dear Peter,

I would like to thank you most sincerely for your enriching book. For five years now the love of the earth has played a central role in my life, but I would never have come across the idea to simply change the way I walk. For a week now I walk differently and can already feel the healing effect considerably.

What I experience in dancing is suddenly so easy to integrate into my everyday life. I believe that there was the desire in my heart to tread lovingly on the earth for a long time, to "dance" on her. And sometimes the heart already knows the way … and led me to myself.

Sincere regards,
Jana, Berlin

Saluti, Peter,

I hold the day under your influence in Lebenskraft in Zurich in good memory and consider myself lucky to have found a further efficient key to the deification of the physical body ("the weakest link"). What I already presumed of you was confirmed in my first experiences (I have already somewhat got used to the image of the "weirdos"), that just like breathing, language, etc., it's about yet another essential, common story, in which we are subject to suffering or to peace, devoid of which further-reaching ambitions would turn out to be flops of the mind. As a person who isn't yet motorised, I now take such pleasure in raising awareness during my kilometres on asphalt, thanks to the automatic heart massage, that it is a joy.

David G.

Hello dear Dr. Greb,

Splayfeet are – beside some other degenerations of the musculoskeletal system – the result of the wrong way of walking.

We have occupied ourselves with optimal foot-related surgical corrections of the de-compensated splayfeet for many years, and have learned with our very successful operative endeavours with the DYNOS-orthopedic foot surgery up until now, that for the best long-term ultimate success, it is extremely important, amongst other things, to bring awareness to walking with mindfulness – in particular with patients affected and suffering from splayfeet; and this already a few weeks before the correcting procedures, then especially postoperative in very dedicated physiological care.

I have noticed that the GODO gait apparently shows some identification with the laws of elasticity and the ballistic of the slanted inclination of the foot, as the last achievement in evolution. But probably due to the unexpected intervention in civilisation of wanting an easy life, it couldn't be provided with that anatomical capacity of stability, that would be necessary to leverage this walking action into a steadfast breakthrough, given all the temptations of civilization.

I take it that you have some tools ready that make the acquisition of the GODO gait easier for learners. I could imagine that for the start – but only for the start – the necessary training of enough stable leg and core muscles and the transformation of the connective tissue, in the sense of installing more elastic components of the "mbt" would be good. For this, the Masai-Barefoot-technology from the Swiss Karl Mueller from the Thurgau region, would be quite a great help.

If you like, I can write more about our discoveries in the operative field of splayfoot surgery, which matches your approach most splendidly. I mostly rely on the physical parameters of classic mechanics and make use of evolutionary biology, biological cybernetics and the well-established causal genesis after F. Pauwels, the orthopaedic father of surgical biomechanics, as "auxiliary science".

With the best collegial wishes,
Dr T. Schewior, Forefootsurgian
drthomasschewior@hotmail.com

Hello dear Peter,

Before I bought your book I had signed up for a walking-course in the adult education centre. Which I then immediately regretted. Well, I thought, paid is paid, now I'll attend it for ten weeks. And now I know why I had to go there. Somehow you always find someone who walks at the same pace. So I always walk together with a woman, to whom I talk a lot. During the first lesson I already told her about GODO. She immediately ordered the book for herself.

Last week, in the fifth lesson, we had to wait a while before we started walking, because a participant was still missing. I made use of this opportunity to tell all the others, including the trainer, about GODO. They laughed a bit when I showed it to them, and then we were all there and we started walking.

Today we were all together again. The trainer said that when she had so many courses, she always had pain in one foot. Now she walked GODO last week as often as she could. And lo and behold, the pain was gone.

Another woman said she had also bought the book. I had a good long conversation with my walking partner. She used to be a gymnast. Now she is the chairwoman of an association for disabled people. As disabled people from the war are all almost "extinct" though, they now do spinal gymnastics in their association. My walking partner runs these courses. Apart from that, she also works with the deaf in the gymnastic field in Zell, Germany. Well, what do you think, she immediately introduced GODO.

Erika B.

Dear Sir or Madam,

I am a GODO fan and always practise it again and again and I'm enthusiastic ... only I have one problem: as a Nordic-walking instructor and a walking-training supervisor (Kneipp society), I should/would like to open up a group and teach them what I do - wonderfully relaxed and easy-going (freshly showered), going up the slowly rising mountain on the partially gravelled forest path in the ball-gait ... I can't and am not allowed to teach it, because I have to demonstrate everything to the people by walking on the heels – and nevertheless I know that it is the right thing to do!

I (born in 1941) have a problem with veins in the left thigh and can unfortunately not practise Nordic walking every day at present, but when I sit, for example in the cinema or at a lecture and I feel an incredible ache, only the ball-gait saves me in the end ... or dancing on the balls of my feet. Or I go for my Nordic-walking in the morning, then only the ball-gait comes in question for me, and I especially enjoy it going up the mountain – this "pull" in the muscles up to the hip-bone. Or in the company of slower people when practising Nordic walking, then I keep up with the increased strain in the ball-gait, because I then become slower. They notice I do the ball-gait as a sensible, effective "in-between".

Could you imagine that we could officially integrate this way of walking into the education of the group? I do this only for myself, as I don't trust myself to pass it on to others, except I would receive the authorization from a competent person, a doctor or an orthopedist.

With kind regards,
Felix Postatny
Vein trainer and Kneipp-teacher (felix@postatny.de)

Dear Mr Biolek,

in your show on 10th April 2001, Peter Greb promoted the ball-gait. Even if it at first sounds a little unconventional that we've presumably undergone an incorrect movement training, many joint and back problems were probably caused by this misdirection. My wife complained about joint problems when hiking, especially when going downhill. Thereupon I practised the ball-gait with her, whereby not the joints, but the muscles and tendons are strained. The success was clear: no joint pain any more.

By the way, this walking technique is what you learn in practising gymnastics, which I did quite intensively in my youth. My meniscus complaints have therefore gotten better with jogging, as I run almost only on the balls of my feet. I could notice that in my footprints in the sand.

The cause of Mr Greb is not exotic in my opinion, but indeed most helpful for many people, if they would only have the right gait training.

But unfortunately, orthopaedics are also not quite taking the right approach, for the strain of the muscles and tendons in the ball-gait is significantly more gentle than the strain on the bones and joints in the heel-walk.

Dietmar R.

Dear Peter,

I've been walking in the GODO way for approximately two months now and have already made such beautiful experiences with it. I am fifty-four years old and all of my muscles are beginning to become firmer again. My scoliosis is beginning to change in the direction "normal" and my hunched back is straightening itself up.

By the way, I sometimes walk barefoot (at home), but mostly in Birkenstock sandals with three straps; I find they are quite suitable for the GODO walk. There are now some with "a soft foot-bed"; maybe this information is interesting for others as well.

All the best for you
from *Marianne Z.*

Hello,

Thank you for responding to my e-mail. I have looked at your website, and a great dam has opened for me. Because I have thought that I was the only one on the planet looking into the barefoot as a way of healing ourselves and thus healing the planet.
You have given me some needed affirmation and I am now in search of your book.

I understand that you have a school?
I would be very interested in knowing more about this.

One of the things that I began to experience as I opened my barefoot back into the forest, learning how to walk ball heel, and then evolving to a grip with my foot as I ran and climb in the mountains, was a growing sense of awareness of the earth. I began to realize that my neural path ways had been cut off.

I have always been interested in training the body, focussing on weight lifting, long distance running and other fitness activities. But as I got up into my forties, I began to have feet, knee and back problems, along with a sense of detachment from the wilderness.
I turned to medical authority to heal me. But none of them could do anything for me. One day while training in old growth forest in the Olympic Mountains, where I am from, I was looking down into a pool of clear water. I had taken off my cloths and I was staring at my body, strong, muscular, full of strength and endurance. Then I looked down at my naked feet and realized that my feet had not kept up with the rest of my body, above my ankles.

The light bulb turned on in my head, and I could see the light.
I wound up throwing away my shoes and going everywhere barefoot, and it was very painful. But I knew that I was right. That I had bought into this cultural mind set of insulating my feet from the earth.
I wound up quitting my job as a heavy equipment mechanic in the city, and returned to the old growth forest in order to learn how to grow my feet. There is no better place to learn how to grow, than in the old growth forest.

I learned that I needed to put four physical qualities back into my feet. These four qualities are motion, endurance, strength and balance. I began to explore many disciplines, and allowed the forest to teach me, the path back to true walk.

One of the techniques that I learned to help me in cultivating my walk and run, is to put stones in my ears, plugging them up, so I can hear the thuds, or the pounding of my feet coming up through my body. I then walk and run on pavement for at least six miles, working on my foot strike, by listening to the vibrations coming through my body. I run until the vibrations are gone, and it is then that my true posture has begun to grow again.

I teach this to many students now.

The thing that is fascinating me now, is the way my sense of awareness is growing, and my sense of touch with the wilderness has opened me up to how disconnected our current way of walking, heel to ball, is separating us from the earth, and throws us out of balance.

I have gone on long enough for now.

I look forward to communicating with you on this subject.

I am currently involved in opening a training centre in the Olympic mountains, that is focused on the barefoot path back into the wilderness, back into our soles, or souls!

Mick The Barefoot

Mick Dodge
barefootsensai@gmx.com

Happy GODO!

"The heel-walk, the heel-walk,
now I declare war to this walk.
The clever one walks on the forefoot,
so that he doesn't have to suffer on foot.
The heel-walk is completely out,
now become a forefoot scout.
The chain of bones are now treated with care,
the muscles do their work I dare.
Then you're quite happy and all right,
you got GODO on your sight!"

Michaela and Mario Reichmann

Dear Dr. Greb,

A friend bought me your book, which I instantly consumed. When I tried this way of walking the first time (for three minutes), my heart chakra opened.

As I am currently writing a book about the new era ("the rainbow era"), I have dedicated a chapter to the ball-gait. As I wrote it, something extraordinary happened, as all seven chakras opened at once, something I hadn't experienced as yet. That showed me that the ball-gait will be one of the most important chapters, or the most important one in the book ...

Apart from that, I have developed a program to open chakras, in which the first exercise is to walk on the spot in the ball-gait. That results in good alkaline quality, which affects the health. I have always wondered why acids pile up in the feet of all places (see also both of my books on acid-alkaline-balance). With your book, my eyes were opened in a literal sense of the words, for with the ball-gait, the acids don't do this any more, no more smoker's legs.

Even my children like the gait; whether or not they become accustomed to it as consequently as I have though, remains to be seen. The ball-gait, due to the shift to alkaline in the pH-value, makes it possible to deal with all the attacking acids much better, and thus with stress and other acid making factors as well.

So how did the heel-walk come about? I believe it was in the moment when human beings started to be in a hurry, and didn't take the time any more to mind every sharp stone, so shoes were invented ... and there were also snakes ... There were probably several more factors which played a roll. Maybe it was the pivotal point in time when we began to eat meat. Meat (and lots of other things) generate too much acid in the body. (Note from the author: fish and other sea-foods, as in our diet during the time when we were aquatic apes, the period of the origin of the people of today, are almost neutral in comparison to meat.) If you start to cleanse the body with fasting and other methods, you will notice at some stage that you can walk barefoot much better. A general transition requires a general change in the way of thinking.

Barefoot-gaiting enables us to absorb the energy of the earth ... through the chakras on our feet. The foot is like the hand, a mirror of the whole body. It has got seven mini chakras, which run in a line starting on the heel (root chakra). By treading with the heel, the root chakra receives a shock. (Many illnesses result from this too.) As a result, the main emphasis lies upon "I am here", on the third dimension and not on "I am" (therefore on our intellectual aspect, which is also present in higher dimensions). Walking in the ball-gait now, the aspect "I am" (crown chakra) is more emphasised and supports intellectual development.

Kind regards,
Patrizia Pfister
papep@gmx.de

On Walking
– Fredrik Vahle –

This literary text from my friend Fredrik Vahle was the introduction in the first four German editions of this book, which was published under the title of *"GODO – Walking with the Heart. The Gait of the new human beings".*

A somewhat strange encounter: a tall person with a long beard stood there and talked about aquatic apes and his own great discovery, about the lost natural way of walking of human beings, which would be good to discover anew and which he called "GODO". Now, what he vividly proclaimed had in no way whatsoever been around for a long time. It's fresher than that, and above all, there's a lot of sense in it. It was after he left the practise of conventional medicine, which had become too limiting for him, that he laid claim to his own life practises. And that made me prick up my ears. Apart from that, I had already occupied myself with the phenomena of "walking", and Peter Greb was thus welcomed with open arms, he didn't even need to kick a door open for me. He was able to step right through it. I also quickly noticed though that after the first euphoric bliss of insight, whole mountains of ingrained conditioning became visible, in the face of which the step back into familiar and accustomed ways of walking seemed to be tempting and apparently natural.

My interest in walking therefore already had a somewhat longer history. It started, amongst other things, with my postdoctoral lecture on the theme of "linguistic creativity". In it I had occupied myself with the meaning of walking for the creation of poetry. For example, an author had voiced: "My poems are made in walking. With the feet on the ground and the words in the head. Out of that came rhythm and finally grammatical form." Or from another one: "compose in walking, write in standing and copy in sitting."

A statement from Federico Garcia Lorca crossed my mind: "The one composes poems whilst walking on her paths, the other composes at the writing desk and observes the paths through windowpanes coated with lead."

And from here it's only a small step to a thought from Nietzsche, which has become more meaningful to us today:

"Sit as little as possible, don't give credit to any thought that wasn't born outdoors and from moving freely, in which not only the muscles are able to celebrate a very special event. All prejudice comes from the guts. Being sedentary is the cardinal sin against the holy ghost."

From this perspective, the history of philosophy can be seen in a new light. Did the main concerns of the early Greek philosophers come into being whilst walking, or in foyers and promenades? Were there then stages in which philosophy sat on its butt and looked at the world through windowpanes coated with lead, e.g. scholasticism? – And then it makes us take a look at the history of religion as well. Were the great religious conceptions of Buddha and Jesus designed in walking, as both were itinerant preachers and roamed around the country on this earth? Is that the movement of transformation? Indeed the life of Jesus, from what we hear, was ended prematurely. Can you notice that in his teachings on various occasions? And yet he has significantly remained the great example for so many meditating people.

I myself had so many difficulties with the sitting meditation: pain in the legs and continuously wandering thoughts. I was made aware of walking meditation a few years ago:

"To find peace nevertheless, you have to be aware of every single step. Your step is your most important activity. It determines everything."

The Buddhist teacher Thich Nhat Hanh said that. And yet that also means that my way of walking has an effect on the world I share as well: I sometimes think that our way of walking, standing, sitting and looking at things has an impact on animals and plants. How many kinds of animals and plants are already extinct because of the damage we have inflicted on our habitat?

The activity of mindful walking was a new approach on meditation for me. It recalled every notion which originated from my ancestors, from the long-legged wandering hunters and herdsmen, who probably all had some difficulties with the lotus position, and who, at the very most knew it as sitting cross-legged. On the other hand, focus on the motoric, psychological side of walking was also brought more into the foreground for me with mindful walking: when the child has matured to the stage of walking, with the movement of the body, the mind also moves, and talking starts. In order to think trains of thoughts, we must first learn to walk. And walking calls again for intellectual stimuli. So it's a switching process. We walk with the legs and think with the head – that can be the other way round in this context: we walk with our head.

The Chinese letter for a "human being" symbolises a person walking.

人 rén human being
入 rù   go inside

Can we still walk mindfully today, or do we only always have to make progress? With energy and a certain defiance, just as we are used to – and that forces us into the heel-walk, or rather it lets it appear to be the only alternative. Maybe this way of walking, which is to be encountered with so-called "primitive people", originates from the Neolithic revolution, when human beings first seized land as their own property, inspected and approved it, walked around it and finally became aware of it. Why should he then still be sensing and feeling it like careful sneaking hunters? One knows one's own property, and one doesn't need to become familiar with it all over again. We know where that leads to. The counter movement to it is regular mindfulness. But even Hugo Kuekelhaus, who had crossed the limitations of the norm in animating our organs and senses with his adventure paths and his thoughts on the terrible neglect of our feet, assumes that "walking is a continuously absorbing issue". That sounds like the perspectives of a heel-walker. At the same time, unintentional mindful walking can definitely take you to your own centre, you can enter inside yourself this way. And that results in a more flowing state of balance.

I clearly felt this flowing state of balance whilst practising a few preparatory exercises for walking in the Feldenkrais method. And moreover, it was determined that such a flexible form of walking represents the original form of dancing. A wonderful experience. And just like all forms of dynamic in walking backwards, crossing over, climbing, creeping, tentatively walking, or skipping works, or rather has to develop into the ball-gait, it was there too. Ball-gaiting appeared to be the natural form of forward motion. And Pe-

ter Greb's great discovery, which actually articulates something obvious, refers to it. But neither Kuekelhaus nor Feldenkrais, nor even most forms of walking meditation, including several ways of walking in Tai-Chi, were able to come to this point. And because of their claims to comprehend the flexibility of all human beings, this is surprising. Maybe the time is now ripe for this in all of the areas mentioned!

The heel-walk is ancient and has spread all over the whole world. It has even begun to take place with primitive people, although the sensitive ball-gait has lived on in the practice of hunters and collectors, in dance rituals and in other dancing forms, for example, in eurhythmics. Due to its spreading and its age, the heel-walk appears to most people as the only rational way of walking. But maybe the same is true for cooking, which radically changes the molecular structure of our food by treating it with heat. Some things which we experience as being quite natural for thousands of years, are perhaps not quite as they seem. Pandora's box, the first cooking housewife in Greek saga, speaks plain language. Meanwhile, lifelong tests and experiments undertaken by Guy-Claude Burger have also brought scientific evidence that life's very good and meaningful with raw, natural food.

Only, what should all the other ones who have set, or have had to set other priorities in their life, say to this? Mindful eating and mindful walking on their own are still no entrance card into paradise, and not even into a meaningful life on the whole. Everyone has other experiences and starting points on their path – be it in the field of meditation, Tai-Chi, yoga, sport, literature, art, religion ... whatever helps people to find themselves, or God on their path. And nevertheless, our intake of food, or such an elementary human mo-

tion as walking, represent fields that are generally speaking of key importance for us as human beings. How easy or how difficult such first steps can become – from our understanding – everyone knows, who has at some time practised a different kind of diet or way of walking, when the social environment lifts its finger (not even the baton) and points to the matter of habit.

Especially in view of these problems, but also because of the magnificence of his discovery, the observations of Peter Greb are so important. They want to give us some courage and not convince us. They show a way to walk, which you can walk with your own feet, in a literal sense of the words. That can mean straightening up, joy and freedom, and such a thing can be transferred onto the world we share.

The Buddhist teacher Thich Nhat Hanh reported that European dogs barked at him when he walked slowly and mindfully. I myself have observed, whilst walking slowly and mindfully in the forest, that foxes and bears let me come up quite close to them, they looked at me and went peacefully on their way. It was as if I was a fellow being and not a potentially dangerous person.

When human beings sat on a horse for the first time, in order not to have to walk themselves, they had problems staying on top. When the first horse powers were produced in a motor car, a servant had to walk in front of it with a red flag to warn the pedestrians. The first cyclists were laughed at. Up until now, humans have discovered means of transport with which he is faster than sound. And he is tempted to fly with the speed of light into space. The own feet fall by the wayside, and the human being has difficulties to understand himself. Is the reflection on something as easy as walking a step backwards the same? Or does the human being have a possibility again for going inside of himself with practical awareness of this way of moving? This new way, rather very, very old way of walking, a more sensitive, and at the same time, a more playful way of walking, is specially a way for men to come out of their rudeness.

Perhaps we can actually start with very simple things now and again. With the way we use our senses, how we lie, sit, stand and ... walk. That such a thing works, despite all these challenges, is a wonderful experience for me. And maybe we really can answer the question "How's it going?" with words that are inspired by happy feet and an open heart: "It's going well. Really well!"

In this sense, I bid this script from Peter Greb a safe arrival into the heads, hearts and ... feet of preferably many people.

Fredrik Vahle, Salzboeden, 12.9.1998
www.fedrikvahle.de

Fredrik Vahle is a private lecturer at the university of Giessen, with the emphasis on language and movement and children's nursery rhymes.

Closing Words

There are many good effects from practising GODO training, but experience it for yourself, take off your shoes and socks and investigate your vivacious feet. Walk in the ball-gait in the rhythm of the motions **resting** to **wanting, thanking, feeling** and **coming-to-rest**. In doing so, tread first of all on the front ball of the foot and slowly come down to rest onto the heel. Enjoy the freely induced, dynamic straightening up of your body posture. Stride through the room with a new feeling and comprehend the words "feel the walking"! Feel into the possibility, ball-gaiting with your toes, that the connecting tissue in your body is unfolding.

Walk simply with feeling, with "loosened chains" and straighten yourself up further with joy, more than the heel-walk allowed you to do up until now. Don't forget about the correct axial tilting of the pelvis, which releases your lower back from the hollow-back posture you had in the old manner of heel-walking. Notice how your breathing has more room, how the breath is felt in your whole body, and enjoy your mood brightening up.

The earth is the lover, the great partner of our body. It is our primary relationship after we are born. We determine our relationship with it in the way we touch it. Whoever realises this, and how much meaning the gestures hold with which our feet nourish the earth, will begin to accept responsibility for every single detail of movement on the ground. Instead of walking on the heels to marching, we will walk with care with loosened feet, hence treading on the forefoot with an emphasis on the balls of the feet. In time we will have freed ourselves out of our prison, meaning from the inflexible manner of the heel-walk.

We will learn to dare to "taper" out of heel-walking conditioning and in doing so we will walk through that invisible gate, which separates the heel-walkers from being aware that the world is paradise.

Our journey together ends here. Now it's your turn! Don't forget: *"There is nothing good, unless you do it."* (Erich Kaestner)

Many thanks to all the heel-walkers, to whom I have also counted myself for thirty-eight years of my life. For without them, or rather without us, this experience would never have been made and this book would never have been written.

With happy feet
and happy GODO

The Training Course to become a GODOLOGIST

The training to become a GODOLOGIST comprises of a curriculum of approximately ninety-hours with holistic medical information and many simple exercises, through which the participant is qualified to walk a path of self-healing and to pass it on to people of all ages in equivalent courses or in private one-to-one sessions.

The curriculum consists of two weekend courses and an intensive seminar of one week, spread over a time of six to twelve months. The starting point of the subject matter is the analysis of the "normal" way of walking and its effects on the body, mind and soul.

Physiological parameters in the circulation, ligaments, connective tissue and nervous system, which change with the ball-gait (GODO), in proportion to the heel-walk, are worked out in detail in a holistic sense. In the process it is medically, psychologically, genetically and morphologically substantiated, spanning from the development of the embryo to birth (regular/water birth) up to the achievement of the erecting of the human being.

GODO is no new theory, no method, but a remembrance of the fact that genetically we are ball-gaiters and not heel-walkers. With the ball-gait we put the heel down after the forefoot in every step.

Topics:

1. GODO, the healthy way of walking and new insights on the development of illness and symptoms.
2. New insights on the development of the embryo and postnatal events, possibilities of postnatal therapy after Robert St John.

3. The evolution of the brain, connections between the development of walking and talking and the meaning of the reptilian brain and the brain stem.
4. Ego-psychology and the development of the ego and the super-ego. What is the ME?
5. The circulation system as our emotional body.
6. Wanting, thinking, feeling – the actions of the spirit with Plato, Steiner and GODO.
7. With comprehensive practical exercises, the participant learns about an ideal ergonomic performance of walking and moving. The value of this is directly experienced in such a perceptible way, that its preventive/therapeutic implementation can be applied in a wide range of fields. A pleasant contribution to it could be GODO water-yoga, guided whilst being moved in water, AQUA-GODO (a training complement, see: www.aqua-godo.de).

Objectives: The participants are qualified to walk a path of self-healing and to pass it on to people of all ages in similar courses or in private one-to-one sessions. They are not therapists. The participants have basic knowledge on a field of associations at their disposal, of the kind that they are inspired to deepen their research on the theme of "healthy walking".

Target groups: Basically everyone is suitable, as previous experience is not necessary. But it is particularly appealing to employees from educational, medical and social fields.

The Institute for applied Humane Morphology
GODO-Walking-school

Information and organisation for the training:

Hans-Peter Greb MD
Beselerallee 46, 24105 Kiel, Germany
Tel.: +49 431/8001501
www.godo-impuls.de
petergreb@godo-impuls.de

Paul Behrendt
AUQA-GODOLOGIST
Seestraße 9, 83209 Prien am Chiemsee, Germany
Tel.: +49 157/89731846
www.aqua-godo.de
behrendtpaul50@googlemail.com

Ellen Schernikau
GODOLOGIST
Bernhard-Kellermann-Str. 34, 39120 Magdeburg, Germany
Tel.: +49 391/617981

Kathrin Schink
TAI-CHI-GODO
Karl-Egon Strasse 15, 10318 Berlin, Germany
info@schink-kantoku.de
www.schink-kantoku.de

And a further fifty GODOLOGISTs, whose addresses can be found on the GODO website: www.godo-impuls.de

Acknowledgements

I would like to thank my friend and publisher Konrad Halbig and his wife Karin Schnellbach, as well as all assistants, employees and followers, for their constant support. And particularly I thank once again the women, and especially my wonderful mother Ursula Reitz, widowed Greb, my spiritual guide Rotraut Mellin for her patient listening and her helpful advice, as well as Ellen Schernikau and Ute Boeters, who also continuously supported me in the turbulent stages of my life.

I'm also a little proud of myself, because I could escape the medical dogma of "decently rolling off", in which I – like everyone else – was pushed into in my upbringing, by false role models and in addition to that by my medical education. Should all those in the medical profession – I have asked myself doubtingly for a long time – not have found it out for themselves?! Consider just how powerful such a comprehensive complete bodily pattern of movement, such as the imitated heel-walk, can banish our body intelligence and our spirits! One can surely be thankful to oneself as well.

Bibliography

Alt, Franz: Jesus – D*er erste neue Mann (The First New Man)*
Ayres, Dr. A. Jean: *Bausteine der kindlichen Entwicklung (The Building Blocks of Child Development)*
Berendt, Joachim-Ernst: *The Third Ear – on listening to the World*
–: *Nada Brahma – Music and the Landscape of Consciousness*
Carroll, Lee/Tober, Jan: *The Indigo Children*
Castaneda, Carlos: *Journey to Ixtlan*
Darwin, Charles: *On the Origin of Species*
Dederich, Markus: *In den Ordnungen des Leibes – Zur Anthropologie und Pädagogik von Hugo Kükelhaus (In the Order of the Body – On the Anthropology and Educational Theory of Hugo Kuekelhaus)*
Enning, Cornelia: *Waterbirth*
Estés, Clarissa Pinkola: *Women who ran with the Wolves – Myths and Stories of the Wildwoman Archetype*
Grof, Stanislav: *Beyond the Brain: Birth, Death and Transcendence in Psychotherapy*
–: *The Adventure of Self-discovery: Dimensions of Consciousness and new Perspectives in Psychotherapy and Inner Exploration*
–: *The Cosmic Game: Explorations of the Frontiers of Human Consciousness*
Hagena, Christian: *Grundlagen der Terlusollogie (The Basics of Terlusollogy)*
Hellinger, Bert: *Love's Hidden Symmetry*
Horx, Matthias: *How we will Live: A Synthesis of Life in the Future*
The –: *Mega-Trend Principle*
Hüther, Gerald: *Begeisterung (Enthusiasm)* (http://www.gerald-huether.de/populaer/veroeffentlichungen-von-gerald-huether/texte/begeisterung-gerald-huether/index.php)

Jung, C.G.: *Das C.G. Jung-Lesebuch* (The *C.G. Jung-reading book*)
Kuby, Clemens: *Heilung – Das Wunder in uns* (The Miracle in Us)
–: *Unterwegs in die nächste Dimension* (Out and About in the next Dimension)
Leary, Timothy: *What does Woman want?*
Leboyer, Frederic: *Birth without Violence*
Liedloff, Jean: *The Continuum Concept: In Search of Happiness Lost*
Long, Barry: *Only Fear Dies*
–: *To Woman in Love*
McDougall, Christopher: *Born to Run*
Morgan, Elaine: *The Descent of the Child*
–: *The Descent of Woman*
Myers, Thomas W.: *Anatomy Trains – Myofascial Meridians for Manual and Movement Therapists*
Nijinski, Waslaw: *Ich bin ein Philosoph, der fühlt* (I am a Philosopher, who experiences)
Odent, Michel/Johnson, Jessica: *We are all Waterbabies*
Orr, Leonard/Halbig, Konrad: *Manual for Rebirthers*
Roth, Gabrielle: Maps to Ecstasy: *Teachings of an Urban Shaman*
Saint John, Robert: *Metamorphose – Die pränatale Therapie* (Metamorphosis – The Prenatal Therapy)
Schernikau, Ronald M.: *Die Tage in L.* (The Days in L.)
Sidenbladh, Erik: *Waterbabies*
Sonnenschmidt, Rosina: *Das Praxisbuch der solaren und lunaren Atemenergetik* (The Practical handbook of solar and lunar Breath Energetics)
–: *Das große Praxisbuch der englischen Psychometrie* (The Large Practical Handbook of English Psychometry)
Steiner, Rudolf: *Philosophy of Freedom*
–: *Eurythmie*

Thich Nhat Hanh: Peace is Every Step – *The Path of Mindfulness in Everyday Life*
Tomatis, Alfred: *Der Klang des Lebens (The Sound of Life)*
–: *Der Klang des Universums (The Sound of the Universe)*
–: *Klangwelt Mutterleib (Sonic World of the Womb)*
–: *Das Ohr – die Pforte zum Schulerfolg (The Ear – the Gateway to Success in School)*
–: *The Ear and Language*
Voss, Jutta: *Das Schwarzmond-Tabu (The Black Moon Taboo)*
Wild, Rebeca: *Raising Curious, Creative, Conscious Kids*
–: *Sein zum Erziehen (Being to Educate)*
Wilk, Erich: Typenlehre – *Magnetismus, Charakter und Gesundheit (Magnetism, Character and Health)*

The author

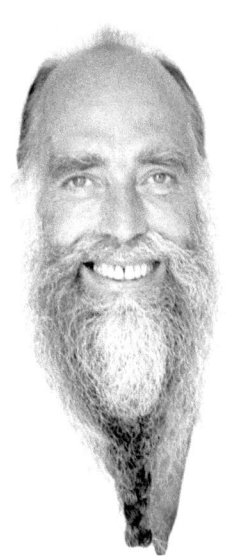

Dr. med. Hans-Peter Greb, observed and investigated the walking pattern of humans during his longstanding practice as a medical doctor and humane morphologist. His uncontradicted scientific finding is:
The human is genetically a ball-gaiter!
With his slogan: »Whosoever once strides, will never march again - GO DO it yourself«, he gently offers the world a key to health and peace.
Dr. Greb explains the issues of the physical, emotional and psychosocial disorders to be seen as originating from the wrong use of our body by walking/landing heel first.

His GODO-SCHOOL of true walking supports a holistic transition, which happens due to the simple and effective change from the heel-walk to the ball-gait. If you, dear reader, would please GO DO it yourself from now on. GODO is just a decision to do good to the world and yourself and thus to become a sound human ...

He runs the "GODO-School of True Walking" under the roof of his "Institute for Applied Human Morphology" since 1979.

He is the author of the trilingual children's book (English, French, German) »GODO - gesund gehen« (healthy walking), GODO Verlag (ISBN 3-9805002-0-9)

www.godo-impuls.com

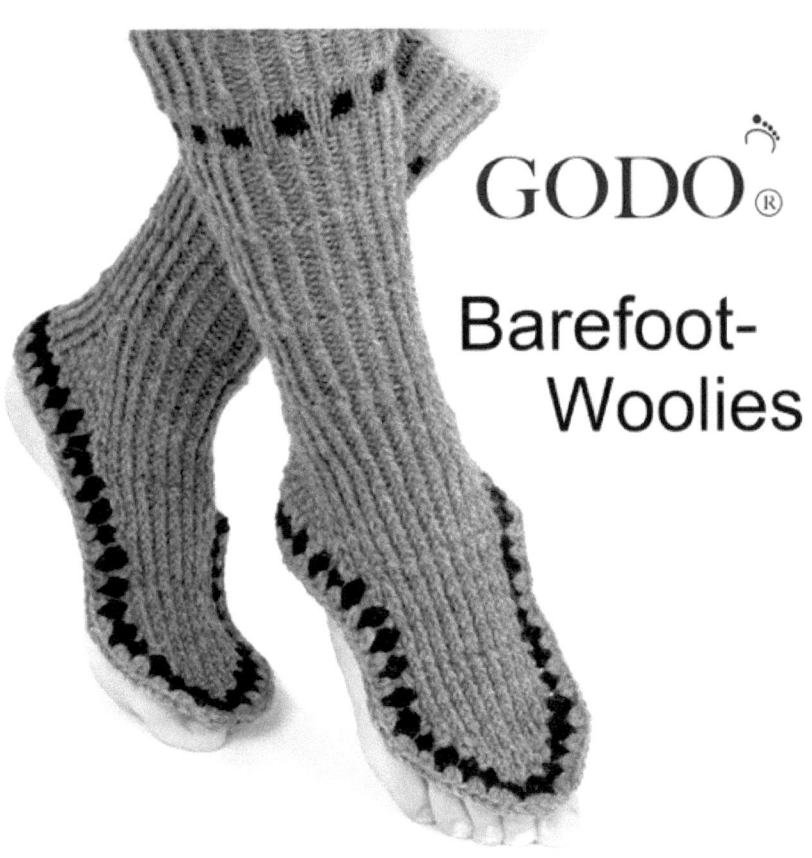

GODO®

Barefoot-Woolies

Ute Boeters
www.fotoatelier-boeters.de
info@fotoatelier-boeters.de